What Else can You Do, but LAUGH?

Christina Luca ADC, CDP

What Else can You Do, but LAUGH?

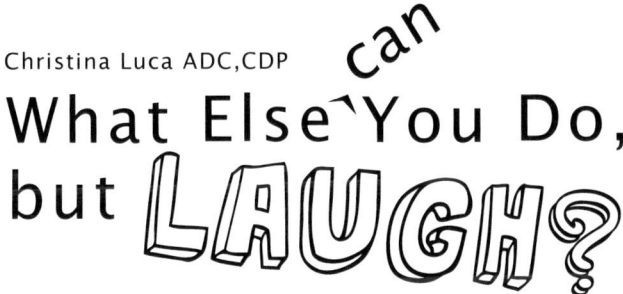

A lighthearted look at the stress and struggles of Alzheimer Disease and Dementia

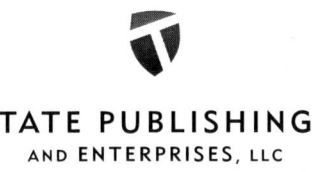

TATE PUBLISHING
AND ENTERPRISES, LLC

What Else Can You Do, But Laugh?
Copyright © 2013 by Christina Luca ADC,CDP. All rights reserved.

No part of this publication may be reproduced, stored in a retrieval system or transmitted in any way by any means, electronic, mechanical, photocopy, recording or otherwise without the prior permission of the author except as provided by USA copyright law.

This book is designed to provide accurate and authoritative information with regard to the subject matter covered. This information is given with the understanding that neither the author nor Tate Publishing, LLC is engaged in rendering legal, professional advice. Since the details of your situation are fact dependent, you should additionally seek the services of a competent professional.

The opinions expressed by the author are not necessarily those of Tate Publishing, LLC.

Published by Tate Publishing & Enterprises, LLC
127 E. Trade Center Terrace | Mustang, Oklahoma 73064 USA
1.888.361.9473 | www.tatepublishing.com

Tate Publishing is committed to excellence in the publishing industry. The company reflects the philosophy established by the founders, based on Psalm 68:11,
"The Lord gave the word and great was the company of those who published it."

Book design copyright © 2013 by Tate Publishing, LLC. All rights reserved.
Cover design by Junriel Boquecosa
Interior design by Caypeeline Casas

Published in the United States of America

ISBN: 978-1-62902-080-8
1. Family & Relationships / General
2. Family & Relationships / Eldercare
13.10.11

DEDICATION

To love someone unconditionally is to love a person with dementia. The pain will fade and your heart will smile when you remember. Honor the person with laughter, with joy, and with memories that will make you giggle.

ACKNOWLEDGMENTS

A huge thank you to all of my friends and my children, Adam and Amanda who have listened to my stories, who have encouraged me, and who have believed in me. To Leslie, first reader who was brave enough and patient enough to correct my spelling and punctuation.

Margaret, thank you for being my second reader and my first editor. God bless each and every one of you.

CONTENTS

Chapter 1:   Going to the village 11
Chapter 2:   Misery Loves Company 19
Chapter 3:   Houdini 27
Chapter 4:   The Answering Machine 33
Chapter 5:   Who Took My Keys?! 41
Chapter 6:   Did He Just Say What I
             Think He Said? 51
Chapter 7:   Was She Talking to Me? 59
Chapter 8:   Has Anyone Seen My Underwear? 67
Chapter 9:   The Aliens Took My Dad! 75
Chapter 10: You Can't Make Me! 87
Chapter 11: Oops, I Did It Again! 97
Chapter 12: Once Upon a Time 105
Chapter 13: Can You Find the Love? 115
Chapter 14: Thanks for the Memories 125

About the Author 129

CHAPTER 1
GOING TO THE VILLAGE

Never underestimate the abilities of someone with dementia.

Marian and her son, Christos, immigrated to the United States in the mid 60's from a small village in Greece. Marian, in her late twenties, wanted a better life for her nine- year-old son and felt the United States would offer him that. After all, the United States had its arms open to everyone. After long arguments with her parents and months of heart wrenching talks with her sister, Marian bought their tickets, she and Christos boarded a plane, and they started their new adventure.

Their first home was a small one-room apartment in New York City, but Marian could only find part-time work. Marian and Christos finally settled in Lynn, Massachusetts. The first order of business was to find an apartment, a Greek church, a Greek school, and work. Lynn had a large Greek population, so they had a ready-made community and felt at home immediately. Marian and Christos found an apartment right across the street from a hotdog factory. The Old Neighborhood Meat Co. made hot dogs, sausage, bologna, and other types of meats. The company had a fairly large Greek population working already so Marian fit right in. Christos was enrolled in Saint Stephen's School. Within a few months, they settled into a comfortable routine which included new friends, steady work, a strong religious community, and a good school.

Marian took great pride in her new life. She also brought some of the things that she liked best about Greece with her; for her that was the Greek gardens. Marian loved to garden. That was her way of feeling like she was home. The more fresh vegetables she produced, the better. She planted and harvested, pickled, canned, and shared with the neighbors. Spending time outside was her solace. It didn't matter what the weather was. Hot, cold, rain, snow—Marian never seemed to mind. Christos would beg her to take the bus when she needed to go around town, but she would just smile, kiss his cheek, and be off. Marian was a kind woman with a warm heart, and everybody loved her.

Christos was a good boy and loved his mother. As he grew, he could see the woman she was and respected her ways. He had been young when he had moved to Lynn but could remember the gardens and villages of Greece, the closeness of the communities, the love of their friends and family, and his mother's joy of being outside as much as possible. He remembered her looking up to feel the heat of the sun on her face and smiling. He knew that she missed her family, especially her sister. Christos knew from the beginning that she had given all of this up for him so that he could become an educated man. His job was to study hard and go to college, and his mother would take care of the rest. They both kept their part of the bargain, and life went on. Marian worked until she retired from Old Neighborhood. Christos went to college, graduated with honors, married and had children. He named his only daughter after his mother.

Shortly after retirement, Marian was diagnosed with Alzheimer's disease. This was a tremendous blow to the family. Christos, remembering all that his mother had done for him, made her the promise that so many of us do: "I'll take care of you; you won't ever have to go into a nursing home." As Marian's disease progressed, her son did everything the right way. Marian's social outlet was the church. He continued to bring her to church as much as possible, but as the years passed he realized that she needed more. He utilized the resources that were available to his mother. He helped her ease into going to a day program. Of course it was a struggle at first. Marian did have a stubborn side. This side didn't come out very often, but it sure came out when it came to the day center. Her only child knew that he had a fight on his hands. After a few arguments and transitions that involved Christos having to go with her for a short time, Marian eased into a routine. She would go for a couple of days a week to socialize and to keep active. This was also a relief for Christos. He could go to work and know that his mother was safe, having a good time and socializing, as she had so enjoyed as a younger woman.

As her Alzheimer's progressed, he had home health services to help with the cleaning and PCA's to help with her personal care. He got her a safe-return bracelet just in case she ever wandered. She loved jewelry so he got her a beautiful bracelet made of gold so that she would be proud to wear it. He had the gas from the stove shut off when cooking became an issue. He had her house checked for safety.

Christos always respected his mother's love for being outside and wanted to find a way for her to continue to go into the yard. Christos worked with the Lynn Fire and Police departments to find a way for Marian to be outside but not wander. It was a learning experience for all involved. He learned the city rules about locking gates, and he registered his mother with the Police and Fire departments. After some time, he was able to develop a plan to have the gate locked, the key hidden, and everything documented. Both the family and the officials felt comfortable with the procedure. This was a good plan and everyone went on with life. Marian went in and out of the house at will. Christos and his family lived two doors down. His Mom went to the day program, the family had dinner together at night, and there were home-based services to maintain her dignity. Christos felt a sense of relief and felt like he could breathe just a little easier. He was right on top of everything regarding his mother's care.

One afternoon, Christos got a phone call from the Lynn police stating that his mother had been found wandering around the downtown area. He panicked and thought to himself, "Downtown, that's two miles away! Oh my God, what happened? The front gate was locked. I check the gate twice a day." He could hear his own voice reassuring himself, "I always make it a point to check every night before I go to bed and every morning before I leave for work. I know that I checked it this morning. The key is hidden, the Police and Fire departments know where it is, but Mom doesn't. Sarah (Christos' wife) locks and unlocks the gate when home services come in. The gate is part of our life!"

He hung up the phone and checked in with his boss to let him know he would be out for a while. Christos made it to the police station within forty-five minutes. He found his mother sitting with a female police officer, having tea and a snack. The police officer had taken off her cap and changed into street clothes because the uniform seemed to make Marian a little nervous. Once she changed her clothes, Marian and the police officer became fast friends. When Christos saw his mother, every emotion that he had came to the surface: anger, frustration, fear, hurt, relief, love, and disappointment in himself. Marian, however, looked at her son, got up, kissed his cheek as she had done when he was a small boy, and offered him some of her snack. Marian had no memory of wandering. In her mind, she was simply having a cup of tea with a friend. As he looked at his mother, he noticed the one thing that Alzheimer's disease couldn't take from his mother. Marian had deep dark chocolate-brown eyes with gold flecks around the pupils. Even as a boy, when he would get scolded for some foolish thing that he had done, he would look into his mother's eyes and see her love for him. With that love he would also see the glint, the smile, and even the playfulness. Her eyes reflected her true self.

Christos had no idea how his mother had gotten out. Contrary to what most of us would do in this situation, he waited and watched his mother. Normally, others would panic and try to fix the situation immediately and usually overreact. He brought her home, and the days went on as usual. One day it happened again. He was in the back of the yard cutting the grass. He couldn't believe his eyes. He held his breath and held back on his basic instinct to run and rescue his mother. He made his feet stay planted where he stood. He wanted to yell. He could feel his chest fill with air but would not allow himself to release the sound. He didn't run and he didn't yell. He watched and waited. In his mother's secure, safe, well-protected world, this loving, faithful son had forgotten one thing. There was a flower pot. Marian took the flower pot, turned it upside down, stood on it and climbed the fence. Marian, in her big house dress, her black stockings, her hair in a bun, and her big clunky orthopedic shoes, was climbing the fence. Again he could hear his own voice, "My mother? For God sake, she's an 88-year-old, short, pudgy, creaky-boned old woman, and she's climbing a four-foot chain-linked fence." The poor man stood there in total disbelief. His elderly mother was scaling a four-foot fence. "What the hell! When I was a kid I got yelled at for climbing that fence." As he walked over to help, a torrent of memories came down on him like rain. Childhood games, holidays with friends, church suppers. The time she had caught him smoking. The beautiful way that she had interacted with his children: the time that she had let his kids play in the mud with school clothes on and tried not to laugh when he got mad about it, the tea parties under the kitchen table on rainy days, getting his kids all revved up at bedtime. He thought about all of the indignities that go hand in hand with dementia. He remembered all of the doctors' appointments and testing. It all came pouring down on him. Then it happened: He found himself smiling. He shook his head and gently helped this stranger that he loved so dearly back onto solid ground. Marian had forgotten how to speak English and had reverted back to the Greek language of her youth, and sometimes even those words didn't make much sense. Christos took his mother's hands in his and asked her where she was going. She leaned forward, kissed his cheek, looked at him with those beautiful youthful eyes and said "I'm going to the village."

The sadness and pain of Alzheimer's is fading for this family. Eighty-eight-year-old Marian, climbing a fence to go to the village, is what her family will remember. Happy, cherished memories are what is important and is what must be remembered. Laughing and loving and passing that on is truly remembering and honoring a person.

Take the time to honor your loved one. What would he or she want you to remember?

Those with dementia never stop figuring things out. When you are a caregiver, you look, you plan, and you think that all of the bases are covered. When you feel that everything is set to keep your loved one safe, look again, and then look one more time.

- Safe-return bracelets can be purchased through the Alzheimer's Association.
- Family members can be registered through the local Police and Fire departments.
- Use your community resources, such as the Adult Day Health programs or Social Day programs, to keep your loved one active in a safe environment.

At one time or another, a physically able dementia patient will wander.

CHAPTER 2
MISERY LOVES COMPANY

Picking a support group is like buying a bra. It might look good and support you for a while, but at the end of the day you feel weighed down and a bit jiggly. It's Time for a new support group

    Ruth and Harry met in 1951, on the very first day of junior high. Harry was a tall lanky boy with curly red hair, big blue eyes, and freckles. Even at the age of fourteen, Harry was on his way to meeting the six-foot mark. His older brother had reached six feet at fifteen years old and was the center for the junior high school basketball team. Harry's plan was to be the next star center for the team and beat his brother's game point average. He had the looks, the height, and maybe even the ability, but the one thing that he didn't have was the confidence. Harry was shy, quiet, and definitely nervous about going to a new school. His older brother had warned him not to tag along. The building seemed much bigger than he remembered from his visit the previous spring. His brother had told him scary stories about the bigger kids, about teachers who would send kids to the office just for fun, and about the basketball coach who made the boys run laps for two hours if they had a bad practice. During the summer, Harry had listened to his brother and laughed at his stories, calling him a liar and walking away. His brother had yelled, "Wait and see!"

Today, on the first day of junior high, Harry wasn't so sure that his brother wasn't telling the truth. With a knot in his stomach and a bead of sweat running down his back, he slowly grabbed the handle of the front door and pulled it open. It was so loud. There were so many people. The teachers were yelling directions. All of the new kids were trying to figure out where to go. It seemed way too much for one fourteen-year-old boy to figure out. Harry suddenly wished that he was back in elementary school. He wanted his quiet, orderly, protected world back. He didn't want to be a big kid anymore. His first day of junior high was going to be terrible. He was scared and he wanted to run, but he couldn't let anyone see how he really felt. He lifted his head, puffed out his chest, and walked through the door.

Ruth was also fourteen. She was the oldest of four children and a whiz in school. She loved to learn and looked at junior high as a challenge. Her goal was to get into college and become a history teacher. She wanted to be the first to graduate college in her family. Her mother and father owned a small hardware store in town and had always stressed to their children the importance of a college education. On the eve of her first day of junior high, Ruth ironed her new plaid skirt and her white blouse. She checked her sweater for lint balls and took out the new black bow from her dresser. Ruth had hoped that she could convince her mother to let her wear a pair of nylons. Her mom would not budge, saying that she was too young. She was also reminded not to wear any of the makeup that she had stashed in her bedside table. Ruth rolled her eyes at the comment and looked over her new clothes one last time. Her first day of junior high was going to be grand. Her bedtime diary entry was full of anticipation and excitement. She was to meet her best friend Peg out front of her house at seven thirty in the morning, and they would start this new adventure together.

Walking through the front door of a new school seemed too exciting for words for both Ruth and Peg. Instead, giggles and audible squeaks came from the girls. There were posters and signs, and for two fourteen-year-old girls, there were boys—"Big boys," not thirteen-year-olds, but sixteen-year-old boys whose voices had changed. Junior high was going to be great!

First there was the confusing task of getting schedules, finding the assigned lockers, and figuring out the lockers' confusing combination locks. Peg found her homeroom with little trouble, and Peg was two doors down. Ruth was where she wanted to be and she was ready for a new year. She looked around the room, trying to see if she recognized anyone. She was hoping that she would know at least one other person. There were no familiar faces.

What she did notice, however, was a very cute red-headed boy sitting next to her. She looked at him and he at her. Neither said a word, but an instant friendship began. Harry realized that junior high wasn't going to be so bad after all. It started with borrowing a pencil from each other. Going to and from school together became a daily event. After the first day of junior high, Ruth and Harry never separated. As they grew up together, they discovered both the good and bad parts of life as a pair. The one thing that was a constant was the special gift of humor that both Harry and Ruth had. In the worst of times, they could count on each other to find laughter. The two dated through high school and college. They had their fights, broke up a couple of times, but it never lasted. They would think of the arguments and realize how silly they sounded. They would forgive each other and move on. Once college graduation was over, the next natural step was marriage. Harry and Ruth built a life together. They raised their children, worked, saved, and talked about when it would be time just for them. Ruth retired from her teacher's post and Harry from his career as a college basketball coach. They were both sixty-five and ready to take on the role of retirees.

    Within two years, Harry and the children noticed some unsettling changes in Ruth's behavior. She became more forgetful and sometimes a little edgy. One Thanksgiving Ruth made tea from potpourri instead of tea leaves. She also tried to use the remote control for the television as the cordless phone. Within the year, Ruth was diagnosed with Vascular Dementia. The news was devastating, but Harry took it as well as he could. He knew his wife and he knew himself. He wanted to understand Ruth's condition, but he also wanted to understand some of the feelings that he had. How would he handle the day-to-day frustrations? What about intimacy?

Harry wanted to learn how to work with his wife through her illness. He didn't know what to do when she got upset. He would try to comfort her in the same way that he had always done. Sometimes it would work and other times it just made matters worse. Ruth sometimes forgot that she had eaten meals. She insisted that she hadn't eaten lunch and demanded her meal. Harry would give her a bit more food because it seemed to settle her mood. Ruth would not accept fruit or low-calorie snacks. She wanted sandwiches or more of a full meal. He knew that giving her extra wasn't a healthy alternative, as she was gaining weight.

Ruth and Harry remained a physical couple even after retirement. Intimacy was important to both of them. Even with dementia, Ruth reached out to him as a wife would reach for her husband. As much as Harry wanted the comfort and solace of his wife, he was no longer comfortable filling that role. He was torn between not wanting her to feel rejected and not knowing how she would accept his advances. Ruth would be playful at times, and other times she seemed to experience mood swings. All of those changes left Harry feeling confused and emotionally exhausted. Every day was an unknown to him. He woke up every morning and looked over at this partner, the mother of his children, his friend, and someone who was becoming a stranger to him.

Harry wasn't comfortable talking with his friends about Ruth's changing behaviors. His friends loved Ruth, and Harry didn't want to mar their opinion of her. But he desperately needed some support. He went to his local dementia resource chapter for a list of support groups. He figured that it would be a piece of cake to find the group that was right for him. He could not have been more wrong. Harry went to what he called a "bereavement group for the living." In this group, everyone told stories and spent the time together crying. Harry found himself looking for the nearest exit and hoping that someone would pull the fire alarm. Another group focused on teaching him all about dementia. He didn't care about what caused the disease or what part of the brain was doing what. He could care less about neurons and brain cells. Harry wanted someone to talk to—to understand how he felt. Another group ended up with two women arguing about some issue that he couldn't even remember. The facilitator didn't seem to know how to get the group back on track. After months of looking, he finally found a group that he felt comfortable with, and he thought that this was finally the one. After the third meeting the group leader called him nightly to discuss his day. He found himself focusing on the hard parts rather than on the happier parts of the day. Though he needed help and support, he also needed to laugh. He needed to tell his stories about his best friend—the person that she had once been as well as the person that she was right now.

Even with dementia, Ruth loved to talk with people and to laugh. When he and Ruth took their daily walk through the neighborhood, Ruth would stop and talk to the children. When they watched television together, she would run her fingers through his curls. Every once in a while she would even become a little flirty. Harry would smile and take her hand in his when she gave him that special little smile. She had the kind of laugh that made you laugh when you heard her. He wanted to share these things about his wife. This was just as important as expressing the sadness that goes with dementia.

After six different support groups, Harry finally found the right one. Yes, there were tears. There was also laughter, story telling, jokes, and a true understanding of what it really means to have a strong support group. During all of the years of the couple's relationship, when things went wrong, Ruth and Harry had a special saying: "Misery loves company." Whatever the issue was, the two would face it together. Harry told the group about that saying. He also told the group that he was glad to share his misery with such good company.

- Get a list of support groups from your local dementia chapter, which you can find on the internet or in phone books.
- Ask the case manager at your local hospital for a list.
- Don't assume that the first support group will be a good fit.

- Be honest with yourself. If you are not comfortable after the second or third meeting, keep looking.
- Bring a family member or friend with you for support.
- No support group should pressure you for donations.

CHAPTER 3

HOUDINI

Even in the best dementia facilities, there are always the one or two that manage to "go over the wall."

I believe that nursing facilities that focus on our dementia population have the hardest job in the world. Each and every staff member has the never-ending task of caring for our loved ones. With love, the specialty staff feeds, dresses, entertains, showers, and pretty much does whatever it takes to maintain a sense of order, dignity and respect for our family members who can no longer manage for themselves. This is a tireless job, and those staff members should be commended for the work that they do.

Specialty units spend a lot of time and money planning for the safety of their residents. Consultants come in and assess the dementia unit. They have their little note pads and pens. They take out the tape measure to get the right size doors and windows.

They look at all of the catalogs to find the latest safety gadgets to alarm the doors. Special lighting is used to decrease sun-downing, and sensors are put under the mattresses to warn the staff of someone who is getting out of bed. Key pads' codes are changed monthly, and even the doors are camouflaged with pretty murals of flowers and birds. Safety is paramount in the dementia unit. You would think that our loved one would be grateful for such loving and thoughtful care. The residents seem happy and carefree. They are busy with daily activities, getting their hair done and living their lives. Dementia units are havens to those with dementia. These have become their homes. So why do they try to escape?

Harold was a gentle man. At the age of ninety, he came to live in the dementia unit of his local nursing home. His children had a hard time leaving him that first day. They waited for Harold to become upset when it was time to say goodbye. In his younger days Harold was a salesman, and he was used to being away from home. Like all of those with advanced dementia, Harold could no longer make the connection that those standing before him were his children. He thanked the friendly people for bringing him to this lovely hotel and shook their hands and said good-night.

Harold shared his room with another gentleman named George. George was a little feisty, at eighty-three. All in all they had a good time together. They went to activities together, watched television in their rooms and could be heard talking and laughing during dinner. The conversations kept repeating, as conversations do when someone has dementia. Harold or George had forgotten what they talked about, so each conversation was new every time it was repeated. Both men seemed happy and content. Family members were pleased with the bond between the two men, and visiting was always a happy time for everyone.

Staff assumed that residents who watch the door to the unit were most at risk of trying to leave. To enter or exit the unit a special code must be punched in. Everyone had to use the code: direct care staff, food service workers, medical staff, family members. It wouldn't matter if the president stopped by. The code was how the door opened. If someone came to the door but didn't know the code a bell was pushed to alert the nurse. Both Harold and George liked to walk with each other in the halls. They strolled side by side, walkers in front of them and baskets filled with things that they found along the way. Some days the baskets held a milk carton. Sometimes it was a little bit of something that they took from the activity room. One day both men had ladies' purses in their baskets. The staff had a hard time figuring that one out. They never seemed to pay attention to the door.

One day the staff had some entertainment come to the unit. Music is extremely important for those with dementia. And this Nursing facility could afford good entertainment. The Activity room was readied, residents came from other floors, and extra staff where brought in to lend a hand. The entertainer played his music and all of the residents truly enjoyed themselves.

George was not really fond of music, so he opted for walking the halls with his walker. Harold noticed his friend and joined in the walk. The nurse kept a good eye on them as she sat at the nurse's station doing her notes. After a few minutes, the door bell rang. The nurse didn't think much about it. She got up, walked down the hall and opened the door. She expected to see a fellow staffer coming to start her shift. Much to her surprise, it was Harold. There he stood with a wide smile with dentures much too big for his mouth. Within a matter of a seconds, the nurse wondered two things. First, how did he get out? And second, whose dentures did he have in his mouth? They most certainly were not his. The dentures had to wait. She had to figure out how he got out. Thank goodness he had rung the bell. Apparently when you have spent your life as a salesman, when you see a doorbell you push it. Within a five-day period, Harold managed to get out and ring the bell three more times, each on a different time of the day, a different circumstance, and with different staff on duty. Harold had the staff baffled. George continued walking the halls with his basket of booty. He would share his treasures with Harold, and the two would have the same conversations over and over again.

One afternoon the unit door bell rang. As the nurse got up to open the door, she witnessed the impossible. As she stood up and looked toward the door, she watched George turn around and push the buttons of the key pad. She watched the door slowly open. She watched a family member come in, and then she watched Harold walk out. How had he learned the key punch? How did he know the order of the numbers? The nurse and her aide just looked at each other. All of a sudden the doorbell rang again. George reached up again and punched in the code. The door opened slowly and there was Harold. Harold pushed his walker to his friend with a big grin. The two men greeted each other as if they hadn't seen each other in years. They sat down, looked in their baskets, and carried on.

- When visiting a specialty unit, be very mindful of codes.
- Remember that residents and visitors can look alike.
- When transitioning a loved one to the specialty unit, discuss : elopement procedures with the staff. (What happens when someone wanders away from the facility?
- There is at least one Houdini on every specialty floor. It could be someone new every day, even every hour.

Direct care staff become woven into the fabric of the residents' lives. Family members look to the staff to keep their family member safe and cared for. Staff members have their favorite stories about residents, as do the families. All direct staff members grieve the loss of a resident just as the family does. Unfortunately, the staff member can grieve openly only for a short time. There are other residents to care for and a shift to finish. When a direct staff member tells a story about a resident, that is a way of honoring that person. Laughter is a coping mechanism for staff members. They recall the humorous antics as well as the more serious moments. Stories help the staff members remember the person, not the diagnosis.

CHAPTER 4
THE ANSWERING MACHINE

Mom's called fourteen times today. It's raining outside, the kids are whining, and you are in a full-blown menopausal hot flash. I bet the last thing that you want to do is pick up the phone and have the same conversation with your mother that you had a half an hour ago.

Martha was a wonderful woman. She had come from Ireland at the age of nineteen. Her birthday present from her parents that year was a ticket on a ship bound for America. She had a small party given by the church, and at five AM the next morning she stood at the docks with her suitcase in hand, waving goodbye to the only life that she had ever known.

She was both terrified and excited. She waved to her parents and five brothers and sisters. Martha had an aunt who had gone to America after marrying a soldier in World War I, who had died in a plowing accident when Martha was very young. From the stories that were told, she knew that the uncle, whom she never had known, had been a strapping, handsome young man. He was tall, blond, and had a sweet singing voice that was admired by everyone—except for the aunt, who admitted that his singing drove her crazy. Her aunt told stories of hiding in the barn just to get away from his voice for awhile. She remembered the day that her mother got the news of the uncle's death. At the time she was too young to really understand what had happened to her uncle. She saw her mother read the telegram and run to the barn to find her husband. Martha remembered her mother being quieter for a few days after that. As Martha grew, she and her aunt wrote letters back and forth. They became very good friends. Martha would share her stories about school, boys in town, about making her own confirmation dress. She would even confide in her aunt when she felt that her parents seemed unfair and treated her like a child. Her aunt would tell her stories of America, about her job and her life.

When her uncle was killed, her aunt had taken a position as a housekeeper and nanny for a young attorney and his family in the Beacon Hill section of Boston. The young family had three children, two girls and a boy. She said that the little boy was a handful and full of the devil, while the girls were both very sweet. Every morning when her aunt went to work, the girls would climb on her lap and give the biggest hugs. With no husband and no children of her own, this was her family.

With much determination, Martha convinced her parents that she should go to America. She would read and reread the letters from her aunt, and her mind was full of pictures and sounds. She could see the colors of the fall leaves. She could smell the ocean and imagine feeling the sand. Her family decided that the aunt would be Martha's sponsor. The aunt would take the responsibility of helping Martha get set up in a job and would look after her and make sure that she had everything that she needed. On her nineteenth birthday, Martha was getting her birthday wish. The steamship whistle blew; she gave one more wave goodbye and felt the vibration of the tugboat pulling the ship away from the docks. Martha watched as her family got smaller and smaller, and then the crowd seemed to swallow them up. She was nineteen and on her way to a new life.

Martha settled in and went to work as a housekeeper for a friend of her aunt's employer. She loved her job, but keeping house was not her life's ambition. She worked hard and saved her money. She loved the idea of being a secretary. She liked the new styles that the Boston women wore, and working in a big office seemed glamorous. Martha taught herself how to type, bought a new dress, hat, and high-heeled shoes, and stepped out into the sunlight. Within a very short time, she had a good secretarial position in a law office. A beautiful young woman, she also had no trouble finding a beau, who soon became her husband. She loved her job and continued working until her first child was born.

As her aunt aged, Martha and her family took her to live with them. The aunt was diagnosed as being senile (the blanket term at the time for senile dementia). Within a short time, her aunt was placed in the local nursing home. As Martha's children grew, she would tell them stories about her aunt's senility and how it frustrated her that she asked the same questions over and over again. The years went on. The children grew and had families of their own. Martha buried her husband after a lengthy illness. He had been in the hospital for a long while, and Martha had gotten comfortable living alone. She had friends in her elderly building complex. She enjoyed the freedom to do as she pleased. Life never stayed the same for very long. However, subtle changes were occurring in Martha, though she did not notice them.

Martha had three children. The two boys had moved out of state, but her daughter, Colleen, who had divorced a few years ago, lived a mile away with her two children, working from home to support the family. As Martha aged, Colleen became her mother's advocate and helper. Martha was diagnosed with early-stage dementia. She had some memory issues but could still live on her own. Colleen had her over for dinner a couple of days a week and send leftovers to be heated up in the microwave. Things worked out fine for quite a while. As time went on, Martha called once a day instead of her usual once every few days. No special topic, she just wanted to say hi. Then the calls came twice a day. Colleen was able to set limits because, after all, she was working. Within three months the phone was ringing four and five times a day. Martha would ask the same question every time she called. She wanted to know where her brown shoes were. Colleen took Martha to the doctor and he explained, "Oh, it's just the dementia progressing. Medically she's healthy; don't worry."

Colleen was a good daughter and loved her mother. She tried to be patient with her mom when she called, but it seemed that every day the phone rang more and more. At one point Colleen grabbed the phone when it rang and, speaking in a stern voice, announced, "Your brown shoes are in the closet!" Unfortunately, the person on the other end of the line was not her mother. At the suggestion of a friend, Colleen got an answering machine to screen her calls. If her mother called and left a message, Colleen could call her back when she had a free minute. Colleen spent a long time explaining how the machine worked, and she and Martha practiced leaving a message. Colleen explained that now Martha could call when she needed to and Colleen would call her back. Colleen was so grateful to her friend. It seemed so simple. She should have thought of that a long time ago. This was a great idea.

Colleen gave her mother dinner, reviewed the answering machine routine one more time, and drove her mother home. During the rest of the night there were no calls. Colleen watched the news and went to bed. At 3:30 AM, the phone rang. Martha was once again in search of her brown shoes. Colleen just sat at the end of her bed, dropped her head and cried. Then she got angry at the unfairness of it all. She got mad at her brothers for not being closer to home. Every time the boys came skipping into town, Martha would be delighted. She treated them like princes. She hugged them, held their hands, and they even took Martha out for breakfast. Martha would tell Colleen all about her brothers. Colleen imagined herself saying to her mother, "Yeah, and you come to my house four days a week. Who takes you shopping, who takes you to your appointments?" She knew that reminding her mother of all that she did would be a waste of time. When Colleen complained to her brothers about their mother's bizarre behaviors, they would look at her and laugh. They would say things like, "That's so funny," and "Oh, Colleen, what do you expect? She's old." Her all-time favorite was, "Come on, it's only a phone call. Just don't pick up the phone." Colleen wondered if solitary confinement in prison would be so bad. If she murdered her ever-patient brothers, she would be locked up, would get three meals a day, and there would be no phone.

Colleen even found herself getting mad at her best friend. Since she had suggested that

Colleen get the damned answering machine, maybe she would give the friend's phone number to her mother. Of course her friend would never speak to her again. So that wouldn't work either. The next morning she declared that she would pick up the phone only twice in a day to receive her mother's call. The answering machine was there to help decrease her frustration.

Technology and dementia do not make good bed fellows. For some of us, technology can drive us batty even without dementia. Martha called, the machine picked up, and then Colleen's fantasy of having a little sanity crumbled. Martha had no clue what to do. Her mother called and talked to the answering machine as if it were Colleen: "Leave a message? But I'm talking to you now. Have you seen my brown shoes? Colleen, are you there? I can hear your voice, why won't you talk to me? Have you seen my brown shoes?" Feeling ignored by Colleen, Martha repeated the litany of questions, just a lot louder. Then she hung up the phone and called again. The whole scenario repeated itself. After a few minutes, Martha spewed out a list of swears and hung up the phone. Colleen was shocked because she never had heard her mother swear. She wished that her saintly brothers could hear her swearing.

Colleen laughed. She remembered all of the craziness that they had gone through. She remembered the bittersweet moments. After all, her mother did like shoes. She sat and thought about her own love of shoes and wondered if someday she would follow in her mother's footsteps. She smiled and picked up the phone to call her mom. The phone rang, Martha picked it up and said hello. "Hi Colleen," her mother said, "I was just about to call you. I haven't talked to you for weeks." Colleen thought about solitary confinement again. But then she realized that however much she hated the calls, someday she would miss them, and the sound of her mother's voice. Prison was going to have to wait.

People with mid-advanced-stage dementia do not remember calling on the phone. Each time they call it's the first time.

- Trying to introduce new technology to someone with mid or advanced dementia is like trying to thread a needle with a telephone cable. Give

yourself a "time out." You can shut the phone off when you need a break.
- Caregiver guilt causes the caregiver to react every time by picking up the phone. Don't feel guilty, you are only human.
- Work with community agencies. There are companion services that can provide activities and stimulation for the person with dementia so that anxieties decrease. It's a juggling act sometimes trying to find the right companion. With some help everyone can have peace of mind.
- Take time for yourself. Stress and exhaustion are the main causes of caregivers getting sick. If you don't take care of yourself, it is very difficult to take care of someone else.
- Do something physical: use a treadmill, walk for an hour, go to the gym.
- Meet or call a friend, someone who will listen and make you laugh—not someone who will say things like, "That's not so bad." Friends are there to make us feel better, not worse.

CHAPTER 5
WHO TOOK MY KEYS?!

Dad is driving to the corner store. He does this every day. He's been doing it every day for the last twenty years. You are getting used to replacing the driver side mirror every time he misjudges the garage door. It might be time to rethink that.

⸻

    If you did a survey asking people if they would rather talk to their teenage children about the birds and the bees or talk to an elderly parent about giving up his or her car keys, I bet you dollars to donuts that talking about the birds and the bees would win, hands down.

    Let me tell you the story of Benny. Benny was a truck driver. He drove a route for a local bakery five days a week for over forty years. He would get up before dawn, grab a cup of coffee, and away he went. It didn't matter about the weather. The only thing that slowed him down were those fun New England coastal snow storms. They slowed him down but they didn't stop him. He drove for a living and he drove for the family. His wife Barbara had never gotten her license. Benny had the same opinion that most other men his age had. He liked his cars to be big. He liked the Crown Victoria and the Caddies. At the age of seventeen he had gotten his license and had driven ever since. Driving was his freedom. It was his livelihood. Driving was his escape. When he and Barbara had a tiff, he would go for a ride. He drove his children to all of their events. When the neighbors saw him driving around town, he beeped the horn and gave a hearty wave. If his vehicle was a castle, then he was the king. He piled the little-league players in the car after a Saturday morning game and headed to the Dairy Queen for ice cream. It didn't matter which team won. Benny and his car took the kids anyway. This was a time before the seat-belt laws. Some readers will remember being piled in the back seat. If there was no more room, you just climbed on someone's lap. Kids laughed, and if a heavier kid got on a skinny kid's lap, then it was even funnier. Barbara found Benny in the driveway on any given Saturday changing the oil, washing and waxing, or with his head under the hood. Barbara was convinced that Benny loved his car more the he loved her. Although at times Benny was a bit of a pain, like most husbands, she was grateful when he would go for a drive. She was even more thrilled when he would take the kids for a ride. It gave her some time for herself.

As in most families, the car was a huge part of their lives. When the car was in the shop, Benny mourned its time away and celebrated its happy return. During his son's painful teenage years Benny used the car as an excuse to talk with his son alone, man to man. The spark plugs suddenly needed to be changed or the carburetor needed to be cleaned. Father and son stuck their heads under the hood, and Benny listened while his son talked about girls, school, sports, and dreams of the future. Under the hood was "for men only."

As the kids grew up and Benny and Barbara aged, little things began to happen. Benny had trouble driving at night. It was a bit of an adjustment, but with a little rescheduling he drove only during the day. Sometimes it became an inconvenience, but nothing major. Again, age snuck up on him. He developed cataracts. First he had one eye surgery to remove the cataract on the left eye. A few months later he had the second surgery to remove the one on the right. Now he had 20/20 vision. Benny was a happy man. He was once again king of the road. He was once again driving his chariot through his kingdom, beeping his horn and waving at his royal subjects. Everything was good in Benny's world. The children called a few times a week to check on their parents, and, after lengthy conversations about anything and everything, the kids went on with their own lives.

On one occasion Benny's son came to visit. He noticed a few little dents and dings on the car's exterior. He also noticed that the passenger-side front tire had a few good-sized rub marks on it. After talking to his dad, he felt reassured. Benny explained about grocery carts in the parking lot, and, oh yeah, he did misjudge the curb once. When the son asked his mother, she agreed with her husband. It's funny how you can notice when something is a little off but you can't put your finger on it. Benny's son was feeling that way. The damage to the car was explained. Mom confirmed it. Benny's son?? had friends in town, and no one had noticed anything strange going on. Dad loved his car. When questioned about the damage, it was as if it didn't really matter. Thinking back, that should have been a red flag for his son. When the boy was young, Benny would have a fit if a stray baseball even rolled too close to the car.

Time passed. A few more dings and rubs on the car, no big deal. Another year passed, and Benny and Barbara got to the point that most of our parents do. They needed a little more help. Maintaining the house was getting harder. Benny didn't really feel safe climbing ladders, and shoveling was too hard for both of them. Sometimes the house smelled a little funny, and as hard as Barbara tried she just wasn't the housewife who she used to be. Benny and Barbara had two children. Their daughter was married with children of her own. Their son was not married, and travel time between work and his parents was only about forty-five minutes. After a family meeting it was decided that the son would move in and help out with the upkeep of the house. He could also keep an eye on his aging parents. Shortly after he moved in, he realized something that floored him. His parents had been declining much more than he had realized. Barbara had a little forgetfulness. Most of her issues had to do with her physical health. She tired easy, didn't eat as much, and was a bit more fragile. Benny, on the other hand, was strong as an ox. He had always been a big man and still carried himself in the same way. His issue was his forgetfulness. Benny would ask the same question two or three times an hour.

His son would become frustrated and Benny could not understand why. He also started walking with a little shuffle. His son was smart enough to figure out what was going on with his dad. Father and son took a ride to the doctor's office, and guesses were confirmed.

This was OK for the son. He talked with his sister and mother. They would work together as a family to help their dad in any way that they could. They all spent some time learning about Alzheimer's disease. Brother and sister did some reading, talked with the doctor, and helped their mother to understand the changes in her husband. They all took one day at a time. They rolled with the punches and got through the day. In his younger days Benny had had a really good sense of humor. This did not leave when Alzheimer's took hold. The family could find a reason to smile almost every day. They were an easygoing bunch, and that style kept them grounded when times got rocky.

On his way home from work, the son saw his dad driving home from the corner store. This was a little unnerving for the son, who had convinced himself it was OK as long as his dad didn't drive very far. He drove to the store. He drove to the barber to get his hair cut. Barbara did the food shopping, and the son took her. All of Benny's destinations were within a two-mile radius. So what could go wrong? He was just around the corner. Benny drove home with his son driving behind him. He stopped at most of the red lights. He only crossed the double yellow line once. He rode with his foot on the brake the whole time. He found his way back home OK. He managed to get the car into the garage, but he left the driver-side mirror lying in the driveway. OK, the light had shined on Marblehead. The two men needed to talk. If someone was going to take the keys, the son wanted it to be him. Benny would understand. He would trust the son's judgment and be grateful that it had come from family.

The siblings talked, argued, and laid out the pros and cons of Dad giving up the keys. This took a few weeks, but in the meantime it was easier to use duct tape to hold the mirror on. It was cheaper and more cost effective than replacing the mirror every time dad put the car back in the garage. In their hearts, they knew that at some point someone was going to get hurt. At least once a month the news had a story of someone hitting the gas instead of the brake. The newspaper ran a story about a car not being put in the park position. Seeing the car rolling down the street and hitting a tree was even worse. The kids finally talked with Barbara and she agreed to stand behind her children's discussions.

It was family meeting time. Daughter and Barbara sat on the couch, Benny grabbed his favorite lazy boy, and the ever confident son took the rocker. Using his calmest voice, the son reviewed the day that he had followed his dad home in the car. He quoted statistics about older people driving. He brought his sister and mother into the conversation. They told him how much they loved him. They didn't want him to get hurt. They asked him how he would feel if he hurt someone else. The children reassured him that when he needed to go somewhere one of the children would be glad to take him. This sounds like a Hallmark moment. The only thing missing was the card. Can you guess what happened next? Yup! You guessed it; the lazy-boy recliner was no longer in the reclining position. Benny was on his feet. He was a good driver! He would never hurt anyone! How dare anyone tell him what he can and can't do? Who were his kids to come and treat him like a child? So much for accepting the news from his son. That pretty much ended the family meeting. Both Barbara and her daughter?? sat crying. Benny stormed off into the bedroom, and the ever confident son just stood there.

When you talk to a family member about giving up the keys, it's always good to have plan B. Benny continued to drive for a couple of weeks. Driving was getting dangerous and something had to be done. When Benny was napping one afternoon his son opened the hood and yanked out a couple of wires that were under the engine. He then called his mechanic and explained about his dad and what he had done to the car. The mechanic was a friend of the family and cared about Benny. He had witnessed the decline in Benny's driving skills. He was more than willing to go along with the plan. Benny went out the next morning. He was going to the corner store as he did every day. His wife watched from the back yard, holding her breath. Benny opened the garage, climbed in and tried to start the car. Needless to say, it didn't start. Benny popped the hood and wiggled a few wires around, but the car still wouldn't start. Benny called to Barbara and she suggested that he call his son. The phone call was made and within an hour the car was towed. After a couple of days the call came in that the car had rusted out from the bottom. Alzheimer's had taken a lot of Benny's short-term memory and some of his long-term. Benny did, however, remember that you should never drive a rusted-out car. The son knew that his dad had a distorted memory around money. It seemed that Benny's mind was in the 1940's when it came to the value of money. His family was counting on this to keep him from getting another car. When asked about a new car, the mechanic quoted a price of fifteen thousand dollars. The king of the road was not going to pay that much money for anything. He called the mechanic crazy and hung up the phone.

Later that afternoon the son came home from work expecting his dad to be angry. Benny told him what had happened with the car. He repeated what the mechanic had said. With a little prompting form Barbara, he was able to tell the son about the cost of a new car. Benny had made a decision. He refused to pay that much money for a car. He walked into the living room muttering that he would go without a car before he would pay that much money. When asked by friends, Benny told them that he refused to pay that kind of money for a new car. Somehow, he felt that it had been his choice to stop driving. It really doesn't matter who did what. What matters is that he is safe.

- Work with the local Registry of Motor Vehicles. State your concerns to them. They will in turn send a letter to your family member and schedule a road test. This is done to test their driving abilities.

- Talk with your doctor. In a lot of cases a parent will listen to a doctor before a caregiver.
- If the parent does give up the keys, take the car off of the premises. Leaving the car in the yard is like having a chocolate cake sitting on the counter when you are on a diet. It's a constant reminder of what you can't have.
- We have all been taught not to lie to our parents. If lying keeps them safe, then the powers that be will understand.
- Taking the keys is one of the hardest things that a caregiver can do. Try not to feel guilty for doing so. Whatever you do, don't give in to the "one more time." The one more time might be the time when someone gets hurt.

CHAPTER 6
DID HE JUST SAY WHAT I THINK HE SAID?

You're a good daughter; you're taking your dad out for breakfast on a sunny Sunday morning, which gives the two of you some time to connect. It is extremely important for people with dementia to get out and socialize.

While you and Dad are waiting for the waitress, you notice that your dad's eyes are following a heavy-set woman as she passes by. He looks at you, and with a fish monger's voice he announces, "Wow! Will you look at the ass on that one!"

Did you ever find yourself thinking thoughts that you know are inappropriate? One example might be: You're walking down the street and a young mother is walking toward you pushing a baby carriage. You glance into the carriage as you walk by and smile at the proud mom. You think to yourself (remember, you are only thinking this), "My lord, what an ugly baby!" But luckily, you know not to voice your opinion.

Everyone knows that dementia is a heart-breaking, devastating disease. People would rather get cancer than have dementia. But maybe there is an up side. If you had dementia, you could say what everyone else was just thinking. At a very young age, we were taught to be polite and mind our manners, especially in public. I remember my grandmother saying to my brothers and me, "If you can't say something nice, then don't say anything at all." Once we learned these rules of conduct, we stored them in little files in our brains. If there was a comment on the tip of our tongues, a little secretary in our brains would run and get the file, open it, and read the file about proper conduct in public. We all learned not to say certain things, but our rules never stopped us from thinking about those things.

A man might say to himself, "My, what a pretty woman." But he would not say that out loud because he could get into trouble. A woman might be walking with her boyfriend or husband and notice him glance her way, yet she would not say something offensive to the other woman. She might just give him a poke because she knows what he's thinking.

Remember the little secretary in our brains, who is responsible for keeping track of our files, also known as our filters. Our filters keep us out of trouble. When a person is diagnosed with dementia, the secretary knows that at some point she is going to get her walking papers. She stays on the straight and narrow for a long time. Then every once in a while she forgets to pull out a file, and the person with dementia says something that should have been censored. A little slip-up, no real big deal. As time goes on and the secretary makes more mistakes, takes more coffee breaks, and does less work, she finally must be fired. People with dementia are left with a jumbled mess of files on the floor. There is no order and no one to keep their thoughts in check, and inappropriate comments are made. Family members and caretakers are embarrassed.

Personalities can also change with dementia. Recently, I talked with a woman who told me that her step-mother couldn't stand her but loved her sister. Their mother had died of cancer when the girls were in their early twenties. Their father had met a woman and remarried a few years later. The step-mom pretended to like this woman, but it was obvious to everyone that there were issues between the two of them. Family gatherings were hard, and everyone tried to work around the step-mother's feelings. The father didn't really notice the tension between the two, or he chose not to get involved.

As an older woman, the step-mother was diagnosed with a form of dementia. As her dementia progressed, her feelings toward the two daughters shifted. The one that had not been the favorite was now the one that the step-mother talked to, laughed with, and enjoyed having around. However, the other sister, originally the favorite, was now cast aside. Dementia can certainly be fickle.

Miss Shanahan loved children, and, from a young age, she knew that she wanted to be a school teacher.

Her father wasn't well, and money was tight for her family, so she decided that she would pay her own way through college. She babysat during junior high and high school, and during the summers she worked at Hoffman's (a department store) in her home town of Lynn, MA. She knew what she wanted and she was willing to work for it. Her mother respected her goal and helped by doling out her chores to the other children so that her daughter could work and save. Miss Shanahan never really had time to date, and the guys didn't understand her drive to work and save. Though she was attractive and sought after by a good number of boys, she dated only every once in a while. She even got engaged once. Her boyfriend had a plan that after marriage his wife would stay home, raise the children, and keep house. Needless to say, the engagement didn't last, never mind a wedding.

She went to a local teaching college in Boston, studied, made a lot of friends, and enjoyed her adventures, but always, her goal was to get her teaching degree, and that's what she did. Her first and only job was teaching first grade at Cobbet Elementary School in Lynn. She started teaching at the age of twenty-two and remained at the same school teaching the same grade throughout her career. She loved everything about her job, the children loved her, and it was within walking distance to her apartment, a small two-bedroom walk-up which she shared with her best friend. The Wonderland Ballroom was in the next town for Saturday night dances, and her church was there for Sunday morning worship.

During the summers Miss Shanahan traveled with friends and explored new places. February vacations were spent in Florida with her girlfriends, and they played golf for the week. Even as her girlfriends started to marry and move away, Miss Shanahan always had a travel partner. She met men, dated, and enjoyed the attention, but her relationships always ended up more as friends than suitors. This would have been an issue for most women of her generation, but it wasn't for Miss Shanahan. After her parents had died, her brothers and sisters remained close, and her children were her students. She loved men and worried about them as if they were her own flesh and blood, but she didn't need or want anyone to take care of her. She loved and was loved. She had a large group of friends and was well respected within the community. She traveled to places other woman read about in magazines, and she had her own money to do what she pleased. With everything that she had going for her, she always valued what her parents had insisted on. She was raised to be a lady. Miss Shanahan could express herself without vulgarity; she would have one mixed drink at a social function but would never get drunk; she dressed as a lady, and she sat like a lady. When she danced, she would never dance too close to her partner. She remembered her father saying, "Leave room for the holy ghost." She was a bit of a prude, but she always had a good time.

Being single and free was how she wanted to spend her life. The down side to being single is that at the end, there is no one to take care of you. Several years after retirement, Miss Shanahan was diagnosed with senile dementia. Her closest friends tried to help her, but the truth was, she needed twenty-four care. She moved into her town's nursing home. It was a good place. The staff was very caring, the food was excellent, and she was able to socialize and have people around her all of the time. She spent hours fussing in her closet, sorting her clothes and rearranging them on hangers. When staff members had a free minute, they visited and engaged in this activity. She shared stories of her travels with her tablemates at dinner and sat on the front porch after dinner when the air was cool. She had many visitors, who brought her treats and flowers, which she always shared with the staff and her friends at the home. It was a good place for her. She was loved, safe, and she felt that she was "home."

As her dementia progressed, her behavior changed. She started to use a curse word every once in a while. This was a shock to the staff, who knew her as always a lady. Her swearing progressed until it was her usual behavior. The staff tried to redirect her expressions of displeasure but found themselves walking away shaking their heads and giggling a bit. Clothes became a bit of nonsense. The staff helped her to dress every morning in a dignified and beautiful way. By lunch time, however, there would be some article of clothing arranged in an inappropriate manner. Her dentures always seemed to disappear, and sometimes she would be sporting someone else's glasses. She blamed the staff for taking her things. She would become angry and then, changing direction, she would sing a song from her youth.

As Miss Shanahan's dementia progressed, the secretary in her brain quit her job. She Shanahan forgot her ladylike demeanor. She forgot all of the things that made her the person that she was. Her new family took over and did what she could no longer do, helping her to be a lady. They helped her get through her moments of anger; they shielded her from her own indignities. They sang the songs of her youth, and they loved her unconditionally.

Stages of dementia are like the seasons. A person with dementia will pass through different seasons, never better but always a bit worse. They have no control over what happens to their bodies or their minds. Love them unconditionally. Find what makes them happy, what calms them; help them in the way that you would want to be helped. What makes them smile today is what will make you smile and remember when they are gone. Miss Shanahan's favorite song was "You are my sunshine, my only sunshine." That song came in handy when the staff needed to toilet her or when she couldn't settle down. The staff and patient would sing at the top of their lungs as they walked down the halls, with staff from other rooms joining in the chorus. Miss Shanahan has long passed, but every time I hear that song I think of her and smile.

- Whether you are a family member or a direct staff member, express your unconditional love toward the person with dementia.
- Dementia can change a personality. Persons with dementia has no control; over what they do or. Or do, try not to get angry with them.

- Think for the person with dementia, there is special clothing that has benn designed to help keep the dignity of the person.
- Keep your sense of humor.
- Ask for help, Use community resources. There are Adult Day Centers that work with dementia in most cities.
- Make time for yourself every day.

CHAPTER 7
WAS SHE TALKING TO ME?

Mom is visiting you at your house. You notice that she keeps turning her head to answer your question. You, however, didn't ask any question. When you picked her up that morning, only one person got into the car. Mom's too old to have an imaginary friend. You think to yourself, "What the heck is going on?"

◦──◈──◦

    Audio and visual hallucinations can be complex and can have several underlying causes. There are billions of sounds around us every day. Noise from television, music, birds and other little creatures chirping, buzzing, and hopping around. The sounds of a busy street. Remember in the good old days when corduroys were in fashion? Everyone knew that you were coming because they could hear the sound of your pants. The clicking of your high-heeled shoes on a cement sidewalk made you feel important. When you got into trouble and your mother said, "Wait till your father gets home," you knew you were doomed when you heard the car coming up the driveway. There are sounds everywhere. There is no such thing as silence., unless, of course, you are on an island in a vacuum. When you are a caregiver to someone with dementia, sometimes being on an island in a vacuum sounds like the perfect vacation.

Sounds can also play tricks on us. You can hear an airplane flying overhead but you may not see it. When the wind blows just the right way you can hear a train whistle blowing from miles away. Rain can sound like steak being fried in a pan. A flag blowing in a breeze sounds like an untied tarp flapping around. Your friend's thirteen-year-old boy answering the phone can sound like his sister. Now add imaginary sounds, or audio hallucinations, and you can imagine what it feels like to be someone with dementia.

Visual hallucinations work the same way as audio hallucinations. Instead of hearing things that are not really there, you see imaginary things.

Any type of hallucination is hard to diagnose. Normally, hallucinations associated with dementia come and go. This makes diagnosing the hallucinations harder: Was a person having a hallucination or did he or she just mistake one sound for another? One of the symptoms of Lewy Body Dementia is hallucinations, both auditory and visual. The early stage of Lewy Body Dementia is harder to diagnose because the patient presents with fewer other symptoms.

Some prescribed medications, over-the-counter medications, and a combination of medications can cause hallucinations. Low blood sugar levels, dehydration, and vitamin deficiency can also cause havoc. The ever famous UTI (urinary tract infection) is one of the primary causes of hallucinations with dementia. A UTI that goes untreated can cause some major medical as well as behavioral changes. To help prevent UTI's, keep that urine flowing. It's better to have to change an undergarment than try to deal with a hallucination.

Connie was a delightful woman. She was born and raised in Marblehead, MA. After her parents died she took over the family bakery. She had two full-time employees to help with the baking and deliveries, and she managed the office. She did all of the ordering of supplies and kept meticulous books, accounting for every penny spent. She was a whiz with money. She didn't need a cash register to figure out what was owed. She did all of the adding and subtracting in her head. Connie fit the mold of the old-time baker. She was short and round; she had the clean starched white apron and the little white hair bonnet. She prided herself on her ability to tie a perfect bow when she wrapped the string around a box of freshly baked goods. She lived only about a half mile from the bakery, so she would get up at four AM, get dressed, and walk to work every morning, seven days a week. She loved her job; it was a living memorial to her parents and she was a huge part of the community. Connie would bake a batch of cookies just to give away. The local school kids would stop by after school, have a free, fresh-baked cookie, and share the tales of their day. For the rest of her customers, she charged a fair price for her baked goods. Enough to make a living and run the bakery, but never so much that she made a huge profit. She loved what she did, and that was good enough for her.

As the years went on and Connie aged, she started to change. There were little changes at first. She was late for work now and then, her apron wasn't as bright and crisp, and she started making mistakes when figuring out balances. Eventually, her employees started to find mistakes in her ordering. They would find the errors and bring them to Connie's attention. She would laugh it off and thank them for all of their help. Her employees were loyal but found themselves covering up more and more of her mistakes. There was one week that Connie forgot to pay them. There were phone calls from her vendors looking for payment for supplies. The community would try to talk to Connie about retiring and taking it easy. They reminded her that she was getting "up there in age" and that walking to work in the bad weather wasn't good for her old bones. Needless to say, Connie wasn't going to give up her family's business. She was on top of everything. The vendors must be making a mistake, because she knew she never missed a payment. Dementia snuck up on Connie, and she could not see her own decline. Eventually, the quality of the baked goods declined and she lost a lot of business. The community felt badly, but they wanted their money's worth.

One early morning in January, Connie slipped on some ice and fell on her way to work. A passer-by saw her out front of the bakery on the ground. He stopped to help and soon realized that she needed to go to the hospital. Connie had a fractured hip and broken arm. She had surgery the next day and stayed in the hospital for a week. The medication that was given to her before her operation caused her to become more confused. Going home was not an option for Connie. After her discharge from the hospital, she went to her local nursing home. The bakery as well as Connie's home went up for sale, and the proceeds helped pay for her care.

Connie became depressed and stopped eating for a few days. With a lot of love and kindness from both the staff and community, she slowly settled into her new life. Friends would bring her baked goods from the local grocery store. Connie would complain about how awful they tasted and that she could tell the difference between homemade and store bought. All of this complaining, however, did not stop her from eating the treats.

Connie's dementia progressed, and the edginess of her first days at the nursing home disappeared. She was a delight. Connie had a good sense of humor; she was pleasant, loving, and carefree. She never gave the staff a hard time about anything. Her nursing home was small and there was time for the staff to do the little extras. One male staff member would take Connie out for a walk in good weather. As they walked around the block, Connie would stop to say hi to a child or pat a dog. Though Connie had never married or had children, she insisted that the male staff member was her son. He never minded her claiming him as her own. In every nursing home there is always the one patient that everybody loves. Connie was the gift that they all shared.

One day Connie asked a staff member to kill the fly that she had seen in her room. She watched it buzz around the room, tracking it with her eyes. She tried to swat it as it flew by but always missed. Connie hated bugs and this was very upsetting to her. In her memory, a fly meant that something wasn't clean. One of the staff members came into the room to find the pesky fly and do it in. No one wanted Connie to be upset. The problem was that there was no fly. Connie pointed it out to the staff, saying "There, see it? It's right there." There was no fly. The staff told Connie that it had flown into another room. Connie was appeased with the story for awhile, but the fly kept coming back. The doctor prescribed something to help her relax. She did relax, but the flies still came back. At first it was only one, but soon there were several. Connie was beside herself and would break out in uncontrollable sobs. The nurse called the doctor and he reminded her that new medications can sometimes take up to two weeks to work. "Just be patient,", he said. The nurse wanted to release some flies in his office to see how patient he would be, but she had no choice but to follow his orders.

Another week passed and Connie's flies continued to haunt her. Now the doctor had the bright idea to test for a UTI. Lo and behold, their poor Connie had a UTI. All of her hallucinations disappeared after a round of antibiotics. Connie was back to her normal happy-go-lucky self. However, there was one strange change in her: She disliked the doctor. No one had ever mentioned anything about her UTI or the frustration that the staff felt waiting for her medication to kick in. She just didn't like him anymore. He would do his rounds and talk with her. She smiled with her sweet smile and answered his questions as best as she could. The doctor would walk away knowing that his charges were healthy and happy. Connie would look at the staff members, point in the doctor's direction, and announce, "There goes a jack ass." The staff would look at her and remind her that he was a good doctor and cared very much about her. Then they would all laugh as Connie just rolled her eyes and shook her finger in his direction.

- When a person shows signs of hallucinations, make an appointment with the doctor. If the hallucinations continue, make another appointment.
- When you suspect that someone is hallucinating, pay close attention to the patient's surroundings. Sometimes patients with dementia feel that the radio or television is talking to them.
- Make sure that a person with dementia is eating and drinking enough.
- Use community services or friends to help out if you are not available.

CHAPTER 8
HAS ANYONE SEEN MY UNDERWEAR?

For some unknown reason, every time you do the laundry you notice that some of your underwear is missing. As far as you know, there are no underwear trolls living in the walls of your home.

One day you see a pair of your unmentionables in your mother's walker basket. When asked, she has no idea what you're talking about. You find yourself in the role of a stalker, tracking your mother's every move in the hope that she will lead you to the hidden underwear.

People become hoarders for many different reasons. There are different types of hoarders. We've all heard stories about the "cat lady," found in some version in every neighborhood. Some people can't throw anything away because they might need it someday. Some might be filling a void in their lives. There are lots of reasons why people hoard.

When a person with dementia hoards, it's not to fill a deep-rooted need or a void in their lives. Hoarding for those with dementia is just picking some things up along the way and then assuming that the object is theirs. In a nursing home setting, a resident with dementia will go into another resident's room and take something. The owner of the property, however, does not take kindly to this. The resident with dementia very rarely wants to give the property back, because he or she is certain of ownership of the item. Then it gets ugly. Residents get angry, the sheriff (the nurse) has to come in and figure out who took what from whom. Feelings get hurt, sometimes there is name calling, and sometimes those old folks can get a little physical. Staff members are really good at working with the residents to get the situation under control. Someone got the bright idea to leave objects out in an open area so that a resident with dementia can fuss with the community objects, thus decreasing the need to go into someone's room to pillage their stuff. A friend who worked in a nursing home told me about one resident who managed to take the strangest things. Staff was always around and she was well supervised. Luckily, she would put everything in one spot, the drawer of her bedside table. Wash cloths, glasses, pens, CNA name tags, silverware, drinking glasses, undergarments, and candy If something was missing, all of the staff knew where to look. It's not easy getting things back from a hoarder with dementia. Compare it to trying to take a baby lion away from its mother. You just can't walk up to the mother lion and say, "Hi, Mrs. Lion, I'm going to take your baby. You're good with that, right?" You would end up becoming lunch. Like any defender of the den, the resident must be coaxed away. Direct staff members are great at this. Redirection is the key when it comes to working with dementia. Some of the staff come in like safari guides in a jeep and lure the resident away. Then others can safely go in and clean out the bedside table and return all of the booty to its rightful owners. It is unfair to upset the resident. She has no idea that the stuff in her bedside table doesn't belong to her. The same methods apply to those living in the community. When dealing with any dementia behavior, kindness, patience, creativity, dignity, and respect will win every time.

From a young age, Hazel was a helper. The oldest of nine children, she was always there to help out her mother and father with chores or her siblings with school work. She helped her friends and she helped her teachers. She even went to nursing school because she wanted to help people. Helping gave her an enormous sense of pride. She worked on the eleven-to-seven shifts at the hospital in her town. No one really liked to work the overnight shift, but that was Hazel's favorite. That shift was a little slower than those during the day, and she could do a little extra for her patients. If someone couldn't sleep, she offered a back rub. When someone was in pain, she fluffed his pillow and sat with him for a little while. When a nurse from the shift before didn't have time to finish stocking supplies, Hazel would finish up for her. Hazel was even nominated for nurse of the year. She won hands down three years in a row.

Hazel got married right out of nursing school. Two years later she gave birth to a baby boy. She lost her husband in World War II, so her youngest sister moved in to help with her son. Working the overnight shift gave Hazel the time that she needed to raise her son and also allowed her to continue doing what she loved. Her sister was wonderful with her son, and they supported each other emotionally as well as financially. Hazel would sleep during the day while her son was in school and her sister was working. She would be up and dressed before he got home. The three of them had dinner together every night. On the nights when Hazel wasn't working her sister would go out with friends or on a date. Hazel had no real interest in finding a new husband. She was happy with her life.

Her son was a fair student. He got through high school but had no interest in college. After hopping from job to job, drinking a little too much, and sporting a black eye or two, he made a decision. This decision was one that his mother had never wanted him to make. He was going to join the service. This upset not only his mother but his aunt as well. The two sisters talked a lot about the service. They both admitted that before Hazel's husband had gone into the service, he was also a bit unruly. Even when he came home from boot camp, everyone had noticed the change. He had settled down. He was calmer, more confident, and more responsible. Hazel could see trouble ahead for her son if he continued going from one go-nowhere job to another. It was a small town and her son was already building a reputation for himself. She and her son talked and she gave him her blessing. She never shared her fears with him. He knew that his father had died in the war. Hazel didn't have to remind him of that. This was the first adult decision that he was making, and she would honor it.

The son with the reputation became a career military man. Like his mother, his passion was to help others, and he found a way to do that by becoming a medic. The service was his life. He worked on medical ships in the middle of the ocean. He worked on land during times of war. He was the one who saved soldiers' lives in the field. Hazel could not have been prouder of her son and wished that his father was alive to see all of his accomplishments. Her son retired from the service after thirty years, and he married and settled in the Philippines. Distance kept mother and son from spending much time together, but they managed to maintain a connection through phone calls, letters, photos, and gifts sent back and forth.

Hazel and her sister continued to live together. They were both happy with their careers and both happy being single. They took care of one another. The two women were sisters, but they were even better friends.

Hazel, the older sister, retired first. She didn't want to, but after years standing on her feet and the physical rigors of lifting and rolling patients, her body was tired. The dampness of the winter hurt her back and hips. Arthritis made her knees swell. At sixty-five she feared the snow and ice. Hazel did, however, volunteer twice a week at the local nursing home. It was easy work. She would sit with one woman who was blind and read the newspaper out loud. She would talk with another who always seemed sad. Volunteering helped Hazel to feel needed and helped the ladies with friendship; they filled a need for each other.

Hazel's sister did the laundry, and she began to find odd things in Hazel's dress pockets—rubber bands, a spoon, an eyeglass case, a roll of white bandage tape. When asked, Hazel had no idea what the sister was talking about. Every time Hazel went to the nursing home, she would come back with pockets full of meaningless things. This went on for a long time. The sister was curious about why her sister had no memory of putting things in her pockets. The sister called a friend at the nursing home in hopes of an explanation. The conversation between friends was uncomfortable and strained. After trying to word her next statement as gently as possible, the friend spoke openly to the sister: "Hazel has been taking things from the residents. We've tried talking with her and it's no use. Hazel gets angry and denies taking anything. We've asked her to look in her pockets and she says that the objects are hers. Unfortunately she will not be able to volunteer anymore." The friend apologized and quickly ended the conversation.

The sister had noticed changes in Hazel but assumed it was just old age creeping in. She was up and down all night. She was much more anxious. Things were missing around the house, too, but the sister had just thought that she herself had misplaced things. The loss of the volunteer job was a blow to Hazel. Her main objective in her life was to help. She no longer had that, and her loss left her sad and unfulfilled.

She would spend hours puttering around the house. The sister retired and planned to watch over Hazel as the two continued to grow older together. The son would visit from time to time, but it broke his heart to see his mother old and confused. The sister was able to keep Hazel at home as her dementia progressed. Home-care agencies helped with housework, personal care, shopping, and companionship. With the help of the home-care staff, the sister collected a box of things that Hazel could rummage through. This was her box. It had photos, soft pieces of material, a ball of yarn, a few hats, and other treasures. The box was filled with objects that felt and smelled good and also held lots of memories. Leaving the box on the dining room table offered something to help Hazel pass the time and decreased the hoarding of other less appropriate things. With a lot of services, Hazel was able to stay with the sister until she passed away.

Decades ago, when the son had joined the service and it was evident that he would not be coming home, the sister decided to keep a journal for him. The journal was filled with the stories of his mother. There were stories of crazy things that the two sisters did together. She wrote stories of his mother and her work. She wrote about the time his mother argued with the Italian woman down the street. It didn't matter to his mother that the woman could not speak or understand English; his mother just kept arguing. She wrote about the time when his mother decided to paint the kitchen. She spilled the gallon of paint on the floor. When it was clear that it could not be cleaned up, she painted the floor too. He had a record of his mother's life. The sister wanted him to remember his mother for the entirety of who she was, not just for the old woman that he saw at the end of her life.

- Keep a box of items handy so that your hoarder can rummage through it at any time. Photos are a great item for your box. Even if the memory of the person is gone, your family member will enjoy looking at them.
- Leave magazines within reach. Like photos, the pictures are engaging.
- Safeguard the house.
- Keep sharp objects and chemicals locked up.
- Get home-care agencies involved. The more help, the better.
- Try not to get angry at the hoarder. He or she does not remember having taken something.
- If you know that your hoarder has something, be creative. Wait until the person is engaged in another activity or sleeping, and then take back your stuff. If the hoarder is holding something, you might be able to trade off with something more inviting.

CHAPTER 9
THE ALIENS TOOK MY DAD!

When the aliens came down, they took "your person," the person that you loved and counted on to be there for you. The aliens left you someone different, someone who is unpredictable. This person is a stranger to your mind and your heart. So, what do you do with that?

⁓⁂⁓

Imagine that you are on vacation. Inevitably, you will forget something in the cottage, but you will also bring something new back home. In your everyday life, not just while on vacation, you are continually leaving something behind and taking away something different. You may not ever know what that something is, but I can guarantee that whatever you take or leave behind, there is a lesson for you to learn or a new discovery for you to make. Dementia takes away the core of our being, robbing families of the loved ones that they knew. When the aliens came to visit, they took away your certainty. In return, they left you with an opportunity.

Frank had always been a hard worker. He was family man and a good friend. He was a Mason, a veteran, and a guy's guy. He loved sports. On Saturday mornings you would find him in his rowboat at the local fishing hole. Sometimes he would take his son; on other occasions it was just for the guys. A rod, a friend, and a couple of beers. Anytime Frank was fishing, it was a perfect day. His wife never minded his going fishing on Saturdays. She would say that Frank worked hard all week, and he deserved some time away. He was always home for supper. He never complained when the kids needed help with homework. On Saturday night he would bathe the kids and get them to bed, and Sunday was for the family. Frank was the best.

Like most of us, Frank had some frustrations in his life. This was the proverbial thorn in his side. The one thing that would send him over the edge was his father. Frank's father, Paul, was everything that Frank was not. Paul was the last-generation father. When Frank was growing up, he constantly heard his father's famous words: "When you live under my roof you will do as I say." Paul was a hard worker, but he drank a little too much. He wasn't an alcoholic, but on social occasions he would have one too many. He would get loud and point out the flaws of his wife and son. To Paul, it was all in good fun. However the comments and remarks left deep wounds in Frank's boyish armor. To protect himself, he went to his room or walked out the back door when his dad started on him. Paul would be quick with apologies. He would grab Frank by the back of the neck, give him a little shake, and say, "I'm sorry, I was just kidding." In his teenage years Frank made himself unavailable to his father. He would go out with friends, go to his room to study, and count down the days until he could be out on his own.

Though Frank loved his father, he never felt the bond that a father should have with his son. When he was young, Frank would ask his father questions: "Daddy, what did you play when you were little?" "What did you do with your father?" "Tell me a story about when you were little boy." Paul would respond, "I'll tell you later, I'm too tired right now." Or "Why don't you go out and play?" Or "Take the dog for a walk." After a while, Frank stopped trying to get close to his father. He figured, why bother.

When his college acceptance letter came in, Frank held it in his hand for a very long time. He ran his fingers over the envelope, feeling every seam and every ridge around the stamp. He held freedom in his hand. In just a few months, he would be in a dorm and doing what he wanted to. He would eat, sleep, study, and enjoy his life. Everything that he did would be on his terms. The "my house, my rule" was gone from Frank's life. The plan was to get through school, get an apartment, and carry on. Frank vowed that he would never move back home after graduation. Home was his past, and the door to the future would be wide open. All he would have to do is to step over the threshhold of his childhood home and leave.

Frank worked all summer, saving as much money as he could to buy dorm supplies and other items for college. Every morning Frank opened his eyes and took a deep breath. Every breath carried the smell of his sweet freedom, always one day closer. Every night he checked the pile of newly purchased supplies and smiled to himself. He was a man, and he was going to live like a man. No more rules, no more guff from his father. All he had to do is stay away from his father and get through the next couple of months.

Frank's mother knew that there is a usually a time when sons don't like their fathers. She had watched this scenario play out with her own father and two brothers. She did her best to keep the peace but also realized that she could do very little when father and son locked horns. Unfortunately, Paul loved his son, but wouldn't show it. Frank didn't understand his father, and as a teenager had no interest in trying. All she could hope for is that with age and distance, the two men would find a common ground. She dreaded the day when her only child was to move away but knew that it was for the best. She wished that her son could see past his father's hardness to the good man that she saw—a loving and caring man and a proud father. : Frank's father would talk about his son to his earned the MVP ring that year and it was presented to him at his baseball banquet.

On the night before moving day, Frank packed his Camry so that he could be on the road early. This was the day that the cage was to open, and he was going to fly. He wasn't going to take time for the breakfast that his mother had planned as a surprise. His mother hid the pain of rejection and walked him to the car. She gave him a hug and he climbed in. His departing words to his mother were, "See, he won't even come to the car

What Else Can You Do, But Laugh?

and say good bye." His father gave a half wave from the doorway and Frank was off. The parents watched their son drive down the street and disappear around the corner. As the wife walked up the stairs, she handed Paul a tissue so that he could wipe away his tears.

Frank spent his first year of college drinking a little too much and sleeping a little too late. His grades were average and expectable for a freshman. When his sophomore year started in a manner resembling the freshman year, Frank was placed on academic probation. Quickly realizing that getting kicked out of school would mean going back home, an unacceptable option for him, he settled down and graduated on time.

As the years passed, Frank went home from time to time to visit. Eventually, Frank and his father did find some common ground. They talked and laughed together. They would have a few beers and watch football. As his parents aged, Frank would help his father with bigger projects around the house. The relationship was never what his mother had hoped for, but it was tolerable The two men in her life had a superficial relationship. Frank never shared much of his life with his father, and his father never shared how he really felt about his son.

Frank married a few years after college. Both parents really liked his wife, and she was good for Frank. Ironically, the couple bought a house only two miles from his parents. On Thanksgiving of the next year, Frank announced that he and his wife were expecting twins. His mother cried and hugged them both. His father hugged them as well and then muttered, "I'm going for a walk." Frank blew a gasket. "See, we tell you guys something wonderful and he walks away." His mother grabbed his arm to make him stop. She wanted to explain something about his father, but Frank was not going to hear it. He grabbed his wife, and then they were gone. Two miles away suddenly became two thousand miles. Frank would give his mother an occasional phone call but didn't want to talk about his father.

The twins entered the world on the first warm day of spring. The little boys were both healthy and grew stronger every day. Frank's mother was allowed to come to the house, but his father was not a welcomed visitor. This was upsetting to both of his parents, but Frank was not interested in how his father felt.

Life went on for both of the families. Babies grew, birthdays came and went. Holidays passed as well as the seasons. Frank's father and mother had always talked about moving to Florida some day, and they thought about it more seriously when Paul retired. They went down to scope out some real estate and came back two weeks later ready to pack. Frank would miss his mother, and the grandchildren would miss their Grammy. Moving day came three months later. The moving van pulled away from the curb, and Paul and his wife headed for the airport. Frank's comment to his wife surprised her: "Now he's out of my life for good." She just let the comment roll off of her back. She had learned a long time ago not to try to defend her father-in-law. She loved her husband and her boys and didn't want to argue.

Three years later, Frank's mother died suddenly from a heart attack. She and Paul had been out for dinner and dancing with friends. She suddenly got winded and had trouble breathing. The ambulance was called and she was rushed to the hospital. She died later that night with her husband by her side. Frank and his wife flew down for the funeral. Frank helped his father with the arrangements and did a few projects around the house. The morning before the flight back, Frank's wife went to the store to get some groceries for Paul. She knew that friends would come by and take him out, but she wanted to be sure that there was food for him. When she was gone, Frank thought to himself as he was picking up around the yard, "He didn't cry when he called to tell me about Mom. He didn't even cry at the funeral. He's a cold-hearted bastard." Frank had had enough. He was done dealing with his father and his "I don't care" attitude. His mother was dead, and his father didn't care. Frank wanted answers, and he was going to get them. It was just he and his old man. Frank opened the shed to throw in the rake and found his father. The cold-hearted bastard was sitting on a bucket sobbing like a child.

Frank froze; he didn't know what to do with this. He was ready for a knock-down argument. He was ready after all those years of cold shoulders and hard-ass treatment to tell his father exactly how he felt. The hard ass picked up his head from his hands and looked at his son. In a voice as quiet as a breeze, he asked his son, "My best friend is gone; what do I do?" Frank turned his face from his father without saying a word and walked toward the house. Paul cried in the shed and Frank in the kitchen. Neither man would let the other see the tears.

After a while Frank went back to the shed. He found his father pulling weeds. He never said a word to his father. He just stretched out his arm and handed him a beer. Neither man mentioned what had happened earlier. They talked about weeds and plants and any small talk that either one could think of. After a few days, father and son shook hands and Frank and his wife flew back to their lives.

Paul stayed in Florida. He went out and socialized with his friends, He seemed OK, and to any outsider it seemed that he was adjusting after his wife's passing. Three years after his mother's death, Frank got a phone call from Paul's friend, stating that Paul was not caring for himself. He wasn't eating. He had stopped going out and socializing. The yard that had been so beautiful was now overgrown and unkempt. Frank had planned a visit in a few months and felt he could wait to assess the situation then. But it wasn't long before Paul's friend called again. He said that when he hadn't seen Paul for a week, he went to check on him and found him sitting quietly. Paul told his friend that he was waiting for his wife to get back from the store. Paul was brought to the hospital, and after a few days of tests he was able to go home. However, Frank was told that his father should not stay alone. He had been diagnosed with dementia.

Frank talked with his wife, and she suggested that Paul move in with them. She was a stay-at-home mom, the boys were in school, and they had an extra bedroom with a bath in the basement. She also reminded Frank that there was no money for a private facility. She was willing to take on the burden. Frank realized that if he said no, then he would look like a fool to his wife and his boys. What kind of message would that send?

Paul's house was sold, and he became the new downstairs boarder. Frank watched his father interact with his family. But the aliens had come and left this stranger behind. This man was not the man that had raised Frank—in fact, he was a nice guy! The kids loved having him around. He was fun. He told jokes, he played with them, and at night he would sneak them candy. He tried to help his daughter-in-law around the house but for the most part got in the way. Frank didn't interact with his father very much. He was polite because of the boys. The twins didn't understand the tension between their grandfather and father. They thought Grampy was "cool." Frank never wanted to share with the boys how Grampy used to be. Every once in a while, Frank would make a snide comment to his father about not having played with him when he was a boy.

As the dementia took hold, Paul would wander. He was found leaning a ladder against his old house, down the street. He had found a gallon of paint in the garage of the old house and wanted to paint it. The problem was that it was not his house anymore and the paint in the can was not the color of the house. Another time he was found pulling flowers from a neighbor's garden, thinking they were weeds. He came home with a puppy once. Frank didn't know how he had found her, but the boys thought it was great. It took Frank a week to find the owners. The neighborhood loved Paul, and people would watch out for him. Most of the time people accepted him, despite their occasional frustration with him. Paul was a happy man. He was safe in the town and he could walk for exercise every day. If he strayed too far, someone would bring him home.

At work, Frank found himself wondering what his father was up to. He would chuckle to himself about some of the things that he had done. Frank found himself developing a soft spot for his father. Paul would drive him crazy at times, but there was less anger and more understanding. Paul could not help himself, and Frank was able to understand that. How could he be mad at his father if he could not understand what was going on? Frank still got frustrated but tried to let it go. He would sit on the front porch with his father at night and have a beer. Paul would tell him stories that never made any sense to Frank. He found himself listening as a child would listen to his father. Paul would be animated and excited with his stories. He would make them both laugh. It was a bittersweet for Frank. The father that he had wanted as a child had come to him when he was a man. Frank would say to his wife, "Why wasn't he like this when I was little?" "Why did I have to wait until his mind is going to find my father?" The only thing that this wife would say was, "At least you have him now."

Paul died in his sleep a year after he had come to live with Frank's family. People stood outside in line to pay their respects at the wake. The whole neighborhood was there. Paul's only brother came with a friend and stayed with Frank until after the funeral. Frank and his uncle talked for a long time one night. Frank asked his uncle why his father had always been so cold to him as he was growing up, why he teased him as a boy, why he didn't even care when he went off to school, why he never had the time to play with him. Why had his father disliked him so much? The uncle sat back and listened to his nephew for a long time. He saw the hurt in his eyes and the pain in his heart. After a long pause, the uncle looked at his nephew and, with a tear in his eye, he touched Frank's knee and told him about his father.

He told him how Paul would call him and brag about Frank:. "He was so proud of everything that you did. High school, the MVP ring, college, the twins. He was so excited when you got married. You were the pride of his life." Frank still couldn't understand any of it. His father had showed no pride, no affection, no love. Frank looked at his uncle for an answer. His uncle looked back at him and explained the reason.

He explained how boys had been brought up in his generation. His and Paul's father would not stand for crying. If you cried, then you were a sissy, a baby, and weak. Crying made you less of a man. His uncle continued, "Your father didn't want you to feel that he was not a strong man. As a child, your father had a sensitive side, a side our father never tolerated. He would hide and cry. I knew what he was doing and so did our mother. If something good or bad happened and the tears would well up, my mother would send him to the store. I would grab him and go outside.

Some people are just criers. He loved you with all of his heart. He just never wanted you to feel that he was weak." Everything made sense now. The times growing up, the announcement of the coming twins, the funeral, and finding his dad hiding in the shed.

- Try to learn about the person's past.
- Encourage expression of feelings.
- Get a feeling of a family dynamic.
- Learn about the culture of the family member's generation.
- Talk with friends of the family member.
- Try to imagine how the family dynamic affected the person with dementia.

CHAPTER 10
YOU CAN'T MAKE ME!

One of the most bothersome responsibilities of a caregiver is hygiene. When you innocently mention that it's time to take a shower, you quickly realize that you've asked the impossible. Every shower day becomes a war of the wills, and the caregiver loses every time.

༺❀༻

Consider yourself lucky if this is not a problem for you. The big question is, "Are they using soap?" How is tooth brushing going? What about the trimming of the nails? Does your dad have unruly nose hair? What about those whiskers that your mom is sprouting from her chin? What about the run-away eyebrows? Are they changing their clothes every day? Hygiene is not just showering or bathing. Hygiene is the whole ball of wax.

Janet was born in France in 1940, the youngest of three children. Her family lived in a small farming community. Her father and grandfather worked growing produce and her mother and grandmother either canned the produce or sold it fresh in the village. Janet had one brother who was two years older than she and one sister six years older. During the day while the family worked, Janet and her brother were under the watchful eye of their older sister. They went to school, came home, did their daily chores, and lived a relaxed and comfortable life. The family unit was strong and based on love and hard work. Though with seven people in the family money was always tight, they had everything that they needed.

As time passed, Janet's grandparents passed away and her mother and father aged. The children became adults and took on the role of caretakers for their aging parents. The three siblings worked hard to keep the farm going. The brother took over the father's role, working the land and growing produce. Having learned a lot from his father and grandfather, he understood the seasons; he understood the growing process and was able to build up a strong, well-maintained farm. His older sister took over the role of the women of the family. She canned, sold fresh produce, kept the books for the farm, and managed the money. Janet's job was to help her mother and father and run the house. Her parents managed for themselves for the most part. Her father had back pain from working so hard as a younger man, and her mother had some memory issues The family continued to work together as they always had. As the parents aged, the children stepped in to help. During a cold, wet winter, the mother came down with influenza. After several weeks, she got better, but the sickness left her weak. Her lungs had been affected and breathing became difficult. The following winter she caught pneumonia and died. This was devastating to her elderly husband. He was no longer interested in the farm. The children could see how much he missed his wife. The doctor tried to help. The father seemed to just give up. When he died, the children and the village people said that he had died of a broken heart.

The son met and married a young lady from the village, and together they ran the farm with the help of his older sister. Janet had been very close to her grandparents as well as her parents. Once they were gone, she saw no reason to stay on the farm. She talked with her brother and sister about her feelings and her need for a change in her life. As hard as it was for them to accept her idea of leaving, they understood. The family talked with a lawyer, and money and property were divided. Janet's brother bought her share of the farm, and Janet had enough money to start a new life. She understood the risks of leaving the family business and loved her brother and sister for respecting her wish to move on.

At the age of thirty, Janet was starting her new life. She had read about Switzerland in her history books and spent hours and hours studying the culture. She loved to ski; she was fond of snow and cool breezy summers. As a young adult she would talk with her father and say that if she could ever live any place besides the farm, it would be Switzerland. Her father would kiss her head and smile. Somehow, she felt better going to Switzerland because she and her father had talked about it so often. Within two months, she was on a plane heading to her new life.

The one thing that became very clear once she landed was the language barrier. Janet was fluent in French and had studied some English while in high school. The language of the Swiss was totally new for her Italian, German? She couldn't even ask for directions on the street. She began to panic as she walked the streets looking for a place to sleep. She held in her tears, but the panic within her chest felt as if someone were beating a drum inside her. Cold sweat ran down her back and she could feel her hands shake. As she walked, looking for a place to stay, she came across a building off to one side of the street. She looked at the sign, and, because it was written in English, she was able to read it: "Rooms for Rent." Under the big sign was a smaller one that said, "Women Only." After a minute or so, Janet noticed that the beating in her chest was a little slower and her hands had stopped shaking. She drew in a deep breath and gave a gentle knock on the door.

The door opened, and, to Janet's surprise and joy, the older proprietor greeted her with a salutation in her native French. She and the matron greeted each other with a familiar kiss on the cheek. Janet asked about a room for rent. The matron smiled and showed her a sunny, well-lit room at the top of the stairs. The two ladies discussed price, two dollars a week in advance, and the rules of the house: "A boarder and a male friend are allowed to sit on the front porch, but never in the house. The front door gets locked at eleven o'clock. with no exceptions. If you are late, you can sleep elsewhere.

Breakfast is served at six-thirty and dinner at seven. No one is to use the kitchen, and lunch is not served. No food or radios in the rooms, and the bathroom is to be shared by all boarders. There is a ten-minute limit in the bathroom, don't leave the water running, and do not hang your wet stockings in the bathroom. If you break the rules, you will have to leave. Do you understand?" Janet smiled and opened her purse, gave the woman two dollars, and put her suitcase on the bed. The woman gave her a half smile and a nod and went on her way.

Janet liked the room. It was filled with sunshine. The white walls made the room look bigger than it really was. There was a twin-sized bed with clean sheets, a dresser with fresh flowers in a vase, and a desk in front of the window. Her new room had an open window with a fresh scent coming in from outside. There was a little wardrobe in the corner for her dress and coat. As she stretched out on the bed, Janet looked around and gave a conscious nod of approval and closed her eyes. She was awakened by a knock on the door. She heard a voice from the other side speaking to her in French. "I have some towels for you." The voice was not the matron's; it belonged to someone younger. Janet flew out of bed and opened the door. Standing there with fresh towels was a younger woman, about twenty-five years old, tall and thin, with wavy dark hair bruched back behind her ears and a beautiful smile. She introduced herself as Demi, and walked into the room and handed Janet the towels. After a brief conversation, the two got their coats and off they went. Demi was going to show Janet Switzerland.

As it turned out, both Janet and Demi had left home to start a new life. Demi had been in
Switzerland for almost a year. She had gotten a job after learning to speak the language. Janet was eager to find out about getting language lessons and getting on with her new life. Demi was a tremendous help, and before either of them knew it, the two had forged a friendship that would last a lifetime. Janet took language lessons, and within a year she found a well-paying job as a translator. Life in Switzerland was good for both women. They had friends, good jobs, and a safe and friendly place to live. Janet was missing only one thing in her life. That was a husband to share it with. She dated from time to time but never anyone whom she wanted to marry. She was now thirty-two and wondering if she was going to spend her life alone. She looked at the matron and saw herself. The matron was alone, grumpy, and spent her time cooking and cleaning for strangers. Janet didn't want any part of that. She wanted a husband, children, and a home of her own.

As part of her job, she was asked to translate for a young businessman coming in from America during his business meetings. His name was Peter, and he was a writer of novels and short stories. He had come to Switzerland on the advice of a friend. Peter and Janet worked together for a week or so before Peter got up enough nerve to ask her to dinner.

They had a good time together; they had a lot in common and felt relaxed and comfortable around each other. Peter made a good living as a writer. He was a kind man with a gentle heart, and Janet found herself falling in love. After working together for six months, Peter told Janet that he was leaving. He had a daughter in America, and his wife had died when the child was very young. His business in Switzerland was winding down and he missed his daughter. On their last date, Peter asked Janet to marry him and come with him to America. She had been heartsick about the prospect of his leaving her. She loved him and he loved her. They got married five days later.

Peter's daughter was a wonderful person. She accepted Janet and the three of them became a family. Their daughter grew, went off to college, got married, and had a family of her own. Janet and Peter settled into the next stage of life. Peter retired from writing and Janet did volunteer work at the hospital. They had a good life, and their love was as strong as it had been when they first met in Switzerland. They talked, laughed, touched, and were the best of friends.

Peter had a stroke at the age of sixty-one. It was a mild stroke, but it left him with some memory issues. He seemed to bounce back quickly and things became pretty normal after a while. On Christmas Day of the next year Peter had another stroke. This stroke again was a mild one. It caused more memory impairments, but he was still strong and could take care of himself. Janet remembered her mother and how her memory had played games with her. Sometimes she could remember and sometimes she couldn't. Time passed and Peter's health declined. He didn't want to eat. He was grumpy most of the time, and he remembered less and less.

A few months after Peter's second stroke, Janet noticed that he was not changing his clothes every day or brushing his hair. She would ask him and he would say that he had forgotten and would laugh. He resisted taking showers. Janet would remind him to shower and he would say that he had already taken one. She would tell him that he was wearing the same clothes and that he wasn't wet. He would look at her, pat his hair, and walk away. Janet found herself sneaking into the bedroom at night and stealing his dirty clothes from the hamper so he wouldn't put them back on. Peter would wake up in the morning looking for his clothes, and Janet would look at him as if to say she had no idea where they could be. This went on for months.

Janet tried to get Peter to shower. She begged, pleaded, got mad, and even called the daughter to see if she could convince him. One morning she got angry and told Peter that she was getting his clean clothes and then he was going to take a shower. Janet got up from the kitchen table to get his clean clothes, and when she got back to the kitchen he was gone. Janet looked everywhere for Peter. Upstairs, downstairs, the basement, the yard; she even called the neighbor to see if he was at their house. She walked up the street and down the street. As she was coming up the walkway to the front door, she noticed something. She looked up to the attic window. She didn't know if she should laugh or cry. Looking back at her through the attic window was Peter. He was waving, with a big smile on his face. When she went to get him, she realized that he had forgotten all about the shower and was just happy to see her. She tried a few more times to get him to shower daily. After a few months she was able to shower him a couple of days a week. Sponge bathing would have to do in between.

Janet realized after a while that if she asked Peter to do something and he refused, she could wait for a little while and ask again. Peter would forget that she had asked the first time and would be more likely to do it on the second request. Life got much easier after that. She never wanted Peter to feel embarrassed. She knew that if he had his own mind, he would be very upset if he appeared unkempt. As hygiene issues came up, she relied on her home health resources to help her with Peter's personal care; she was happy to give that duty up to someone else. Janet realized that Peter responded much better to a man when it came to showering and hygiene issues, so she made sure that her home health aide was male. His male aid talked of current events, the sports page, and his children. The aid was quick and respectful, winning both the trust and friendship of Peter.

- Be patient when asking someone to accept help with hygiene issues. It takes time and trust. Remember that we are taught as children not to take our clothes off with a stranger. If a person with dementia doesn't recognize you, then you are a stranger.
- Try offering a shower. If the person refuses, wait and ask again later.

- Use home care agencies. Let them handle hygiene issues. It will decrease the frustration between you and your loved one.
- Communicate to the person. Tell him or her what you are going to do. Not knowing can be frightening.
- When you are showering a loved one, start from the feet and then go up.
- Keep the bathroom warm.
- Have conversations while you are showering your loved one. It will keep him or her occupied.
- Good hygiene is extremely important. It is essential for good health.

CHAPTER 11
OOPS, I DID IT AGAIN!

When a person continually repeats the same question, it can make you want to pull your hair out in frustration, yet this person is not really trying to drive you crazy. He truly doesn't remember asking the question before.

When a person repeats a behavior over and over, it's not that she is trying to get you to jump off the proverbial bridge. The behavior is all new to her. She doesn't remember doing it before.

Sam was one of five boys, the middle child. He always felt that he was too young to be with his older brothers and too old to be with the younger ones. Sam had a loving and supportive mother and father. His parents worked hard and provided a good life for their boys. They had a good-sized home and enough land to keep five boys busy. The back yard had a big oak tree for swinging. There was a hitch-and-post fence for climbing and enough space to handle the endless energies of five boys.

All five boys had a knack for building, and there was always something being built or torn down. There were forts, tree houses, club houses, or bike ramps. Five boys and their imaginations could dream up just about anything. Their parents saw their love for building and always kept enough supplies on hand to feed their little builders' dreams. As the boys grew, tree houses turned into drama sets for school, storage sheds, rough furniture, and cabinets. All five boys went to the local trade school in town. Each had his own specialty, but all of them studied some type of wood shop. Two brothers studied cabinet making. Another learned to custom build furniture. Sam and his younger brother opted for construction. As the boys turned into men, they realized that within their own family they had the ability to build homes, furnish them, and design hand-made cabinetry and kitchen layouts. With the financial support of their parents, the boys opened their own family construction company.

The business grew and prospered, as the young men worked hard to build the trust and respect of their customers and their community. They were honest; they would go above and beyond and never went back on their word. Because of their company's reputation, the boys never wanted for work. In the winter, orders where filled for furniture and cabinets. In the spring, summer, and fall, homes were built. As the years went on, all five boys married and had children. The company was solid and continued to grow. It was hard at times, but rewarding as well. Each family member was able to raise his family comfortably as the result of his labors.

What Else Can You Do, But Laugh?

Life was good for the family, and as one generation grew older, the younger generation stepped in. It was a family-owned business in every sense of the word. Family members ran the show from payroll to plumbing. All outside sub-contractors were hand picked and supervised. The brothers had an excellent reputation.

Sam headed the construction end of things for the business. He drew up blueprints, got city permits, found sub-contractors, and did most of the behind-the-scenes work. He also did the hands-on building. He loved being outdoors, no matter what the weather. He didn't mind the heat in the summer but hated the rain, which meant no construction work for that day. Sam loved the work, but what he loved more was watching his children and his nieces and his nephews. He watched them grow, learn their trades, and step in to keep the family name alive. He was especially proud of his daughter. At sixteen, she announced that she was going to become a plumber's apprentice. In 1951 that was quite an announcement, unheard of at that time. His daughter worked hard. She accepted all of the teasing and the rejections from the boys in her class. She didn't care; she knew what she wanted, and after a few years she earned her master plumbers license.

As Sam got older, he felt the aches and pains of the construction business. Arthritis took hold of his back and knees. His hands and arms hurt most of the time. On cold days the dampness would settle into his bones. At the age of seventy-five Sam decided that it was time to retire. Like his older brothers, he was given a lavish retirement party at the Lions Club, with lots of love, laughter, friends, and family, and a big check for $5000, to be spent on whatever he wanted.

As Sam settled into retirement, he enjoyed his grandchildren and his friends at the local diner. He quickly built a routine for himself. He took his wife out on Sunday afternoons for a drive. The two would always find a nice place to stop for lunch. He started to enjoy all of the things that he had missed when he was a younger man and the family business had taken up so much of his time. He joined the local bowling league on Thursday afternoons and had a few beers with his sons on Saturday nights.

Sam was a healthy man. Other than his tired old bones, he had no other diseases or physical problems. Sam never smoked, he drank moderately, and his wife always made sure that he ate right. As a construction worker he could vent his frustration, stress, and anger out on banging nails.

At the age of eighty-two, Sam started repeating himself, and his wife became concerned. She would answer his questions, but within a short time he would ask again. She took him to the doctor and had his ears checked, but his hearing was fine. She also noticed that Sam went to the cellar a couple of times a day. She asked what he was doing down there, and he replied that he was cleaning his tools. She didn't think much of it, as he had always kept his tool box clean. Soon, however, he was going down to the cellar four, five, or six times a day. He would go down, putter around, wipe down his tools, and come back up. Sam's wife talked with her children, and they agreed that if it made him happy, then "What's the big deal?" When his subterranean forays increased to as many as ten times a day, his wife was getting extremely concerned. He started leaving the supper table to go to the cellar. He would get up from watching the television to go to the cellar. Once while he was in the shower he got out and went to the cellar. His wife found him coming up the cellar stairs with nothing on. Before she had a chance to say anything, Sam looked at her and said, "I think the furnace is broken; it's cold in here."

Another trip to the doctor confirmed dementia. Sam's wife talked to her children and explained their dad's condition. Everyone pitched in to help. The kids took turns hanging out with their father. One son would take him out for breakfast once a week. Another would take him to work and let him hang out in the tool shed. The sons put a second railing in the cellar stairway for Sam's safety. Home services were brought in to give his wife some time away. She had two hours three times a week to visit friends, get her hair done, or do some shopping. It was hard to leave Sam at first, but she got used to the idea and then started to look forward to her "own" time. With everyone on board and a little help from some medication, Sam's world was well planned and safe.

However, though Sam was safe, his family had a very hard time dealing with his behavior. He continued to go up and down the cellar stairs, and now it was almost non-stop. It got to the point that he would walk up the cellar stairs into the kitchen and then turn around and go right back down. Sam's wife got so frustrated with her husband that she would just sit down and cry.

Finally, one of the children put a lock on the cellar door. Sam's tool box was brought upstairs and left on the dining room table. This way Sam could take care of his tools all day and not go down to the cellar. It seemed like the perfect plan. When Sam went to the cellar door, his wife would remind him that his tools were in the dining room. Sam didn't seem to mind. With the cellar door locked and the tools on the table, Sam's wife relaxed and the house was a calmer place. Everyone was happy.

One night Sam's wife woke to find Sam missing from their bed. She looked for him all over the house, until, as she rounded the corner to the kitchen, she got the shock of her life. The cellar door was open and the lock was on the kitchen table. She went down the stairs and found her husband sitting on his stool cleaning his tools. He greeted her as if he hadn't seen her in weeks. When she tried to talk to him about the locked door, he had no idea what she was talking about. She sat with her husband for a long time until he finished cleaning. She watched the way that he moved; she noticed the size of his hands. She looked at his face. She could still see the young man that she had married. This was the man who had worked so hard to build a good life for his family. She missed that man. After a few minutes, Sam put down his rag and took his wife's hand. He couldn't find the words that said "I love you," but she felt his love in his touch and could see his love in his eyes. Her husband's mind was disappearing, but he still loved her. This was a moment that she would hold onto for the rest of her life. For just a little while, nothing else mattered.

Sam's wife called her son the next morning and recounted his father's escapade of the previous night. The family was bewildered; they couldn't figure out how this could have happened. How could a man with dementia have remembered how to unscrew the screws to get the lock off? One of his sons got an idea. He put the lock back on and relocked the cellar door. He asked the rest of the family to leave the kitchen and sit quietly in the living room. Sam sat at the kitchen table with his son drinking a cup of coffee, something they had done for years. Sam's son finally stood up and asked his eighty-four-year-old father with a diagnosis of dementia to help him take the lock off the door. Much to his son's surprise, Sam took the screwdriver from his son and went to work taking off the lock. He handed the lock and all of its pieces to his son and laughed. The son just shook his head and laughed with him.

As the family investigated a bit closer, they noticed little things that were not quite right anymore. The batteries to the remote control were missing. The knobs on the china cabinet were missing. Photos that hung on the walls of the spare bedroom were now missing as well. It seemed to the family that Sam had been working around the house for a while before the cellar lock incident.

Sam lived comfortably for another six months before being placed in a local nursing home. He settled in quickly and finished his life's journey with his wife and family by his side. Sam's antics are still talked about with his family. There is a running joke that when something is missing, everyone says that Sam is fixing things again.

- If you have to put a lock on a door, place it above or below eye level. People with dementia tend not to look up or down.
- Keep tools and sharp objects away from someone with dementia.
- Don't assume that putting something in a drawer will keep it hidden.
- Assume that someone with dementia will revert back to his or her old job or old habits at some point.
- Recruit home care agencies as much as possible.
- Keep familiar objects around so that your family member can use them safely.
- Remember your loved one's past experiences to predict his or her future behaviors.

CHAPTER 12
ONCE UPON A TIME

When working with a person with dementia, putting yourself in their "present" can be extremely difficult. You could be anyone—a brother, sister, father, mother, the milk man—who knows?

As a person's dementia progresses, lots of different things happen. In the earlier chapters we talked about cognitive changes causing problems such as hallucinations, repetition, personality changes, hoarding, and many other issues. I think that when the person that you love loses all memory of you as a loved one, it's the hardest road for any caregiver to walk. You spend your whole life knowing someone, and at some point you either become a stranger or you become someone else altogether, often someone else who is significant to the person with dementia.

It is very common for a husband to become a father to his wife or a wife to become a mother to her husband. Remember, short-term memory goes faster than long-term memory. Remember the secretary in our brain? Every day when she was working, she would spend time moving older memory files way to the back of the file cabinet. Memories of a childhood got pushed back to make way for newer memories. As memory fades away, the most recent memory goes first. That's why someone suffering with dementia can't remember what he had for breakfast but can tell you a story about sledding down a hill when he was twelve. When your person with dementia loses you and you become someone else, try to have patience. Your person is not trying to be mean or hurtful. That part of his memory is gone. It's not because he wishes it to be that way; it just is. All you can hope for is that you become someone that your person liked in the past.

I'll tell you a story about one little Jewish woman, a Holocaust survivor, that I worked with in a day-treatment center. This story might be a bit upsetting but it will tie a lot of different dementia issues together. I've worked with many dementia patients in my over thirty years in direct care But this one afternoon opened my eyes to a world that I had never seen before.

My little friend Bertha was about seventy-five pounds and about four-feet-nothing tall. She was a tiny little lady with a lot of spunk. She lived in Swampscott in a small assisted living facility. The bus would pick her up three days a week and bring her to the day center. She had one daughter, who was very supportive and loving with her mother. Bertha's husband had long since passed.

As a child, Bertha and her family were caught up in the Holocaust. She was able to avoid going to the concentration camps, but the rest of her family were not so lucky. After the war, she ended up in New York. As a young woman, she worked in the fashion industry. She loved her job and made a good life for herself, working hard but also enjoying herself. She went to dances and parties. She had a wonderful sense of humor, and everyone who knew her loved her. She was never at a loss for a date and enjoyed the respectful affections of her suitors.

When she got married and settled down, she and her new husband stayed in New York for many years. They both continued to work and raise their baby daughter. Life was good for Bertha. She felt safe and secure living in the city. Her tenement had young families like her own. Everyone watched out for one another's children. There was always someone to talk to or gossip with. Bertha put her past behind her and was a happy, well-established woman with a good life. On hot summer nights, the children got their baths and were put to bed. The adults would spend long hours on the front stoop trying to catch a breeze. They would talk, laugh, and enjoy each other's company. Life stayed this way for many years.

As the years passed, families moved out of the neighborhood and went on their way. Times were changing in New York City, and the secure world that Bertha and her friends had created was changing as well. Families had worked and saved. It was time to leave the city and head for the suburbs. Long-time friends said their goodbyes and wished each other well. There were promises to write and visit one another. Bertha and her family joined the exodus from the city and headed for the ocean and Massachusetts. They settled in Swampscott, a small, quiet town, but one that was growing. The town's people welcomed the newcomers. Swampscott had a strong Jewish community, and the synagogue was the arm that wrapped itself around its community. It seemed that there was a new family moving in monthly. It didn't take long for the family to settle and find their way. Bertha and her husband bought a home, their daughter was enrolled in junior high, and new jobs were found within a week. Swampscott served as a playground in the summer. On a hot day everyone was at the beach, and at night there was almost always a breeze. The winter chill off of the ocean could bite sometimes, but it was tolerable. Swampscott wasn't far from Boston either. Shopping in Boston was a favorite pastime for the women, and Boston was close enough to go to a show on a Friday night. It was a good life for a long while.

Several years after they had moved to Swampscott, Bertha's husband passed away from a cancer. It had been a long illness, and Bertha was as prepared as any wife could be. He was buried in the ways of tradition, within twenty-four hours of his death, and before sundown on Sabbath, eve, and Bertha and her daughter sat Shiva (the Jewish period of formal mourning) for seven days. Bertha's husband had saved during the years, and with his pension Bertha and her daughter had a nest egg. Bertha continued to work because she wanted to, not because she had to. She paid her daughter's way through college, and when her daughter married Bertha was able to give a gift of a down payment on a home for the new couple.

Bertha's son-in-law was called to another part of the country for work, and his wife followed her husband. Bertha missed her young family, but she was comfortable in Swampscott and she didn't want to move again. She had her work, her synagogue, and her friends. Bertha continued to work until she was sixty five, and then she happily retired and enjoyed her new freedom. She played cards with her friends, shopped when she wanted to, and truly was at a place in her life when she didn't have to worry about anyone or anything except her own well-being.

Yup, you can guess what happened next. Bertha was diagnosed with dementia. She declined at a slow but steady pace. No great catastrophes in her life, no sickness, just a slow, predictable decline. Bertha slipped comfortably into her dementia and never really noticed when it happened. With help, she was able to stay home for a long time on her own. She had help with meals and housekeeping. She had a companion to take her out to eat or to go shopping. Her friends continued to visit and take her out. Even as Bertha's dementia progressed, she continued to live and love her life.

Eventually, Bertha went to one of the local senior day centers. She enjoyed being at the center. She had a great sense of humor and an easy friendliness, and the staff and the other clients loved her, and she loved them. She brought joy to the hearts of everyone that she touched.

After a while, Bertha began to become more confused, and her present and past became more and more intertwined. The past that she had tucked so deep down inside of her mind began to emerge, not all at once, but in pieces. She would hear a noise that was not there; she would complain of an awful smell. There was nothing that anyone else could hear or smell. And after a while she began to become resistant to using the ladies room.

On one particular day, Bertha refused to go into the restroom, which she had used hundreds of times before, seeming to feel comfortable and safe when staff brought her in. On this day she flat out refused. She cried and pushed and pulled away from staff. She tried to leave the building, and she reverted back to the Yiddish of her youth. All of these behaviors were uncharacteristic of Bertha, and the staff couldn't figure out what had happened to get her in such a state. Nothing had changed. The day was the same as any other day, the staff was the same, she had been in a good mood all day; none of us could figure out what had triggered such a change in her behavior.

Within a short while, Bertha settled down and was back to her old self. She joked with staff, talked with her friends, and ate her lunch. We took a collective breath and just kept an eye on her. After lunch, Bertha needed to use the restroom again, but as soon as she started to walk through the door, the behaviors started again. She cried, kept saying no, and kept pushing away the staff. We decided to help Bertha by giving her a portable toilet in the privacy of the nurses station. She went in and did what she needed to do. We realized that it wasn't the act of using the toilet, it was the restroom itself. The staff went into the restroom to try to look through Bertha's eyes, but they couldn't see anything unusual about it. They thought for a long time and kept looking. Suddenly, one of the staff realized something. The floor was white, the walls had been painted a light blue (people with dementia can't distinguish between light colors, so the walls looked white to her), the ceiling was white, and there were no windows.

Bertha had escaped having to go to the concentration camps as a child, but sadly, her parents and older brother hadn't. Bertha had heard stories about the war from survivors and imagined the horror that her family had had to endure. In her mind, the restroom had become a gas chamber. The thought of Bertha's terror devastated all of us. How could we not have seen that? Why couldn't we as the staff have put two and two together? I went into my office and cried; I could only imagine what her mind was going through. This was unacceptable, and all of the staff had to figure out what to do.

At the time, a local store was selling pictures that looked like windows. The pictures had outdoor scenes with shutters on either side. One was a beach, another was a woodland scene, and another was a garden. We bought the pictures and hung them in the restrooms. We also had recordings of relaxing sounds that seemed to make the pictures come to life. After we had put everything together, we held our collective breath. When it was time for Bertha to use the restroom, I think that you would have heard the proverbial pin drop. Staff went into the restroom, flipped on the recording, and invited Bertha to come in. She walked in and spent her time in the restroom talking about the sea gulls on the beach. It had worked; with a window, Bertha didn't feel trapped. The relaxing sounds were familiar and reassuring to her. She knew that the staff members where her friends and she was safe. Bertha would sometimes have other flashbacks. We as her caregivers learned what would trigger them and how to help her through them.

Bertha spent two more years with us. She devoted herself to the task of fixing up the staff with each other. The staff were all women at the time, but in Bertha's mind someone was always a boy. She could be fresh sometimes and say little "dirty" remarks about the staff. We had a couple of Yiddish-speaking participants who would find great joy in translating for us. Bertha spent a lot of time loving the staff and accepting love back from us. Whenever I think about Bertha, I am reminded that I always have to look, listen, and never assume that I have all of the answers. Everyone with dementia is an individual. Their stories are all different, and their past is their own.

- If you work in direct care, learn as much as you can about a person.
- Remember that everyone has a personal story.
- Talk with families to get a family history.
- Watch for triggers (something that causes a reaction). Some triggers are good; the smell of food can bring back a pleasant memory. The sound of a gun—even on the television—can trigger a bad reaction in someone who was in a war or was exposed to other violence.

- Try to see a situation through the eyes of the person with dementia. Remember that our five senses play a huge roll in understanding the life of someone with dementia.
- Always watch and listen; as dementia progresses, a behavior can appear where there was no behavior before. If a new behavior develops, always seek medical counsel (remember the UTI).
- Use the people around you to brainstorm. Sometimes someone else might be able to notice something that you've missed.
- The goal of working with someone with dementia is not to make you feel good. It's to help your person get through the day feeling safe, happy, loved, cared for, and respected.

CHAPTER 13
CAN YOU FIND THE LOVE?

Your anger, frustration, tiredness, and impatience cannot be hidden under a bushel. You may be sporting that cheesy smile and speaking in your favorite sing-song voice. Guess what? A person with dementia can see through your façade. While she may not know exactly what's going on, she knows that something's up.

⌘

 The old expression "poker face" might ring true in the old western movies, where the grimy cowboy would win a hand of poker just by looking angry and staring down the other grubby guy across the table. His eyebrows would go up and his forehead would get all crinkled. Everyone who was watching the movie knew that he was bluffing, but because this was a movie, the poor slob on the other side of the table never had a clue. If you try to pull a fast one on someone with dementia, chances are that he or she will be much more observant of your body language than that "other grubby guy" in the movie, and you won't succeed in fooling anyone with your poker face. Body language is an amazing thing. Did you ever walk down the street and see an old guy with a scraggly beard walking toward you in a wobbly line? His speech was slurred and he didn't make much sense. What did you do when you came across this man—even though he might have been a perfect gentleman and a loving grandfather of twelve? You reacted, your shoulders dropped, you looked away, and you may have stepped off to one side. The message that you gave to the old man was "I'm very uncomfortable right now."

Lucile Ball did a movie for television about twenty years ago. In the movie, called "Stone Pillow," she played a homeless older woman. During one of her breaks from acting she went to get coffee and visit with the people on the streets.

She stayed in costume as she approached a group of women. Even though the women knew who she was, they backed up because of the way that she looked; they would not make eye contact. All of this happened in a matter of seconds, but it was long enough for Lucy to watch their body language. You can tell a lot about a person by the way they move, the tone of their voice, how they direct their eyes, even how they sit. You don't have to hear the words to read a person.

Remember when you were a kid and you did something wrong? Your parent or teacher would say, "Look me in the eye." You did everything short of putting your head in your pocket not to look your accuser in the eye. Your person with dementia is going to look at your face. They are going to watch the way you handle yourself. Is my caregiver angry? She is smiling, but why is she tapping her fingers on the table. She is speaking to me in a gentle voice, but why is she being so rough with my tee shirt when she's folding my laundry? Your person can also feel your vibes.

Did you ever have an argument with someone, and afterwards, sitting in the same room makes you feel uncomfortable? Neither one of you is speaking, but you just want to head for the nearest door because you are emotionally uncomfortable. In most situations, a person can figure out why he or she is feeling uncomfortable. Put yourself in the shoes of someone with dementia. He sees you, he hears you, and he reads your body language. He is feeling uncomfortable in his own skin, but he doesn't know why.

Ester had two sons, both raised the same way, taught the same values, sent to the same school, and put in a shared bedroom until they moved out as adults. Ester and her husband had a stable marriage, and they were together until Ester's husband died in his seventies. One son grew up and became a brick layer, working outside building walls, chimneys, and patios. He worked hard. He married, raised his family, and did what he needed to do to keep food on the table and a roof over the heads of his family. The other son joined the service right out of high school. After he was honorably discharged, he went to college. He graduated and became a lawyer. He too married and raised a family. He had many difficult cases and worked long hours. He had a nice house, fancy car, and vacationed with his family every summer. Both men loved their mother and helped her whenever she needed it. The sons would cut the grass and fix whatever was broken. She could count on them for whatever she needed. Either son would stop by on his way home from work to check in, and mother and son would have a cup of coffee and talk for a few minutes.

Parents say that they love all of their children equally, and I'm sure that they do. Most families, however, have different relationships with each family member. If you come from a bigger family, you may have a brother or sister who is your favorite, more like a friend than a sibling. When you are together, your body language says that you are happy, relaxed, and comfortable. With another sibling you may sit a little straighter, be a bit more guarded in conversations. It's just what you do. You are not consciously guarded; it's just the way it is.

As Ester aged, she needed more help. She became frail, didn't eat as much, and became more forgetful. The sons never complained when their mother called. They would make time for her; after all, she was their mother. She had been there for them, and they would be there for her. Ester had a series of TIAs (mini strokes) during the first part of the New Year. Because of her TIAs, her forgetfulness turned into dementia. Her sons understood what the doctors had told them. It was decided that Ester would stay home for as long as she could. She loved her home; her memories lived there with her, and she felt happy and safe there. Both sons lived close by and felt confident that they could handle things as they came up. Home services came to prepare meals and to do the housework. A personal care attendant came to help Ester shower, and a companion

What Else Can You Do, But Laugh?

came twice a week to take Easter to lunch or get some fresh air. Everything ran like clockwork. When a problem did come up, one of the sons was right on top of getting the problem solved.

Ester's memory continued to decline, and she had a harder time remembering her sons. She knew them from somewhere but could not remember that they belonged to her. Both sons continued to be good sons in spite of their mother's memory loss.

When the son who was a lawyer came to visit, he would always come in, kiss his mother on the top of her head, and go to the kitchen to make them a cup of coffee. The mother and son would sit at the kitchen table and spend a little time together. He would ask her what she had had for breakfast even though he knew that she couldn't remember. He would get up and look in the refrigerator and pantry to make sure that there was enough food for meals. He brought the daily newspaper and would thumb through it as he talked to his mother. Ester always seemed to get a bit restless after about half an hour. Her lawyer son could never figure out why she would get fidgety and seem to avoid looking at him. He would ask her if she was alright. He knew that her answer would never come, but he always asked. After a few more minutes, he would always say the same thing: "Mom, you must be getting tired; I'll leave so that you can rest." He would walk her to her sofa and help get her feet up, cover her with her afghan, and kiss her on the top of the head. He always checked his watch before he left. He knew that the home service worker would be in within the hour to make her meal. He was a good son and truly loved his mother.

On other days her other son, the brick layer, would come in to check on her. He would come in the back door instead of the front. He would always call to his mother while he was taking off his brick-dust-laden shoes. He would head straight for the coffee maker and put a fresh pot of coffee on. As he talked to his mother he would wash his hands and pour two cups when the coffee was done. The mother and son always sat in the living room, the mother in her rocker and the son on the sofa. He would put one leg on the coffee table and one arm over the back of the sofa. He would tell her about his day. He worked hard and would share some of the crazy things that he had seen while he was working. As he told the story of his day, he would laugh. He told her about his wife and about her grandchildren. He told her that he couldn't decide who was worse, his son who had decided to paint the dog or his daughter who did nothing but whine. Easter would rock and listen. She would throw her two cents in even though the words didn't make sense. Her son would look at her and say, "I know what you mean," and laugh. He would stay for about an hour and then get ready to leave. He would take the cups to the kitchen, and he always left a little snack and a glass of ginger ale. He would say, "Just in case you get hungry." He knew that the home care worker would be in to make sure she ate, but it was just something that he did. He would kiss her on the head as she walked him to the door.

The brothers would always check in with each other after their visits. The lawyer would say that his mother seemed a little tired, and the brick layer would always say that she was in a good mood.

Even in her dementia, Ester was a happy woman. She didn't suffer from depression and was quite healthy for a woman of her age. She stayed home for about a year after her diagnosis of dementia before being placed in a nursing facility. She felt comfortable thinking that her new home was her old home. She had people to talk with and things to keep both her mind and body busy. It didn't matter that her dementia had gotten worse; she could still love and be loved. The staff took good care of her and met all of her need in a loving, kind way.

Her sons continued to visit almost daily. Sometimes Ester would become withdrawn when her lawyer son came to visit. She seemed happier after a visit from the brick layer son. The staff at the nursing facility took note of Ester's reactions to her sons. Both sons loved their mother and treated her gently and kindly. They brought her gifts, and on holidays the sons would bring her home for a few hours.

After a while, the director of social work called the brothers in to discuss Ester's care plan. (A care plan is a list of goals and objectives that the facility puts into place for the next 3 or 4 months. All of the facility's disciplines contribute to a care plan—nursing, OT, PT, activities, speech therapy, and any other services that a person might need.) The facility and family review the care plan before it is put into action. During the conversation about the care plan, there was a discussion about Ester's different reactions to her two sons' visits. The director of nursing was a kind young woman who cared very much about her patients and was a bit baffled by Ester's reactions after visits. The three talked for a long time about the visits and tried to figure out what might be different about each son's visit.

After a long time and several more visits, one of the staff noticed the difference. When the lawyer son visited, he spoke very quietly; he sat on the edge of the chair and asked her questions that she no longer understood, or he moved around the room and seemed not to be relaxed. When the brick layer son came in, the room was full of good energy. He was relaxed, animated, and told his stories but didn't ask many direct questions. Both sons loved their mother and she loved them. Neither son did anything wrong, but they had different personalities and demeanors, and Ester felt more comfortable with one of her sons than to the other. If Ester had been someone else, she might have been more comfortable visiting with the lawyer son. We all react to body language, to non-verbal communication, and to our gut feeling. When someone has dementia, in most cases this doesn't change.

After the staff discussed their observations with the lawyer son, he paid more attention to his body language. He stopped asking direct questions and instead told more stories. He also stopped moving around the room and sat next to his mother or directly across from her. Ester could see his face when he spoke. Visits became pleasant for both Ester and her lawyer son. The sons visits continued until Ester passed away two years later.

- Pay attention to your facial expressions and body language.
- Make eye contact with a person with dementia.
- Don't ask direct questions if they have trouble processing what you're asking.
- Watch the ways that the staff interact with your loved one; they have a knack for finding what works.
- If you are uncomfortable visiting, bring a photo album and show family photos. Even if your loved one doesn't recognize the people, he or she will usually enjoy looking at the photos.

CHAPTER 14
THANKS FOR THE MEMORIES

You've walked down such a hard road and you've muddled through. You don't know how you did it, but you did. You've gotten angry, you've cried, you've run the gamut of emotions. You've been robbed of your person, the one that you've loved and taken care of.

Your life has been a series of twists and turns. You've been spun around so many times you feel like you can't even walk straight anymore. So what do you do with that? What do you hold on to? With everything in life there is a choice. You can hold on to the pain, anger, and sorrow or you can find the love and the laughter. It's your choice.

I'll bet that every one of us has had a loss. Something or someone in our lives that was important to us has been taken away. Someone may have lost a pet. That loss can be catastrophic, no matter what someone might say if they don't love animals. A person may have lost a loved one, and there is no doubt that is catastrophic. It doesn't matter who or what was lost. Your loss is a hole in your heart; it's a part of your life that is now missing. I don't claim to be a psychologist or a counselor, but I can tell you that I've seem my share of loss. Working in direct care pushes death to the forefront of your life. With elderly people, there are two things that you can count on: One is that at some point they will lose their dentures, and the second is that they will die.

Sitting in a room that is so very quiet with a patient who is passing is both the worst and the most treasured moment. There is no better gift to a person who is dying than the gift of love. I sat with my first dying patient when I was fourteen. I can still see the room; I can still feel her hand in mine. Her aged hands were so soft, like chicken bones wrapped in silk. The nurse asked me to sit with her while she brought medication to the rest of the patients on the floor. Then she was going to sit with both of us while the woman let go of her life. At first I was terrified. I went into the room and stood in the doorway. The old woman seemed so small. I didn't realize at the time, but while I was standing in the doorway, inside of me something begged me to go closer to her. I pulled up a chair very close to her bed. I found myself holding her silken hand and comforting her. I talked to her in the hope that somehow she could hear me, I talked about the weather, and I just talked. It was so comfortable. I found that I was no longer terrified but had found a peace in my own heart that I'd never felt before. I could only assume that she felt the same kind of peace that I was feeling. It didn't seem that her passing took a long time, probably no more than an hour. When she passed, I heard a noise in the doorway. When I looked up, the nurse was different. The shift had changed and I'd been sitting with my lady for over four hours.

Apparently the nurses would pop their heads in to check on me. I never noticed. I was busy making sure a special person was being sent on her way. Her name was Sarah Kennedy and she passed away at the Alba Nursing home in Lynn, Massachusetts. When a person with dementia is on her journey home, it's a long slow walk. She sheds parts of herself along the way. All of the things that were learned along life's path become discarded along the side of the road. The little things go first, and then the bigger things. Through the years, her load gets lighter. She has less to carry, less to worry about, and less to burden herself with. There are no pressing issues of the day and nothing that needs her attention. When the time comes to end her journey she is freed of everything that she's learned. She is are "truly free." There is no pain, no suffering; there is just sleep.

The person with dementia gets the easy part. She discards what she's carried for so long. The caregiver is the one who has to walk behind the person and try to pick up everything that she's shed. The caregiver's arms get heavier and heavier until they feel like they can't possibly carry anything else. Somehow, the caregiver gets just enough oomph to carry that one more thing, which feels as heavy as a boulder. The caregiver carries on.

We have choices in our lives. We can choose what we want to keep and what to throw away. You as a caregiver can't possibly hold on to everything. Think of your person's heart as a gift to you. When you open the gift, you get rid of the wrapping paper and keep what's most important. The gift that you find inside contains all of the happy, funny times and the crazy moments that your person with dementia has left you. Throw away all of the stuff that isn't important—the wrapping paper—and cherish the gift.

- Find a support group that fits your needs.
- Use your local resource center to gather information about dementia chapters in your area.
- Don't isolate yourself from friends and family.
- Share the stories that make you laugh. If you find a time when you can't laugh, someone will remind you how.
- Keep a diary; write down only the things that your person did that made you smile.
- Remember to keep your load light. Get rid of the stuff that is weighing you down.
- Let people take care of you; if a friend asks you to go to dinner, say yes.
- Remember to honor those you have worked with, carry their memories in your heart, and share their stories.

Thank you for allowing me to share my stories with you. I will continue to honor those who have touched my life. They've taught me the important thing. They've taught me the true meaning of love.

ABOUT THE AUTHOR

Christina Luca has worked in direct care for the past 38 years, specializing in dementia care. She started working with the elderly at the age of 14. She has worked as a PCA/CNA, Activity Director, Staff Development Coordinator, Hospice Care Provider, Support Group Facilitator, Mentor, Corporate Consultant, and Volunteer coordinator. She is also a Nationally Certified Dementia Practitioner and trainer with the NCCDP (National Council of Certified Dementia Practitioners) as the president and owner of C. A. Luca Dementia Consulting, an Alzheimer and dementia educational service.

Working with those with dementia has given me a gift that I can never repay. I've been given the gift of love. People with dementia don't care how much money you make, where you live, what you do for a living. No concerns about the car you drive or the size of your house. Those with dementia have taught me that all of those things? don't matter. What really matters is the ability to love unconditionally, to respect, to care for, to cherish every day, and to honor our elders, to keep them safe, and to always remember to laugh.